BEYOND THE MAGIC BULLET

Also by Bernard Dixon

INVISIBLE ALLIES

JOURNEYS IN BELIEF

WHAT IS SCIENCE FOR?

Beyond the Magic Bullet

by
BERNARD DIXON

HARPER & ROW, PUBLISHERS

New York, Hagerstown, San Francisco, London

For Jacqueline, James and Stuart

FIRST U.S. EDITION

ISBN: 0-06-011062-7

LIBRARY OF CONGRESS CATALOG CARD NUMBER: 77-11811

Contents

Acknowledgements

Many people, in many different ways, have contributed towards the genesis of this book. In particular, though, I would like to thank for their help, Katherine Adams, Mike Bessie, Jon Evans, Paul Harrison, Peter Leek, Mike Muller, Patricia O'Flanagan, Ian Porter, Lewis Thomas and Geoff Watts.

I
A beguilingly simple idea

A beguilingly simple idea — so obvious to modern eyes that its historical emergence seems to have been agonisingly slow — has dominated the growth of modern medicine over the past 100 years. That idea is specific aetiology — the notion that particular diseases have particular causes. One man, Girolamo Fracastoro, glimpsed this truth around the year 1540, but his name does not appear in this book because, being far ahead of their time, his speculations had no tangible influence on the evolution of medicine. Specific aetiology really took off with the discovery of 'germs' a century ago. Since then it has permeated, with dazzling success, most other branches of medical science and practice. Yet today that same notion, when applied to coronary heart disease, much mental illness, and indeed most ill health throughout the world, seems to have lost its explanatory power and potency. So, in mid-1977, we find an international medical journal, *The Lancet*, airing a debate centred on the fact that doctors no longer even agree on what they mean by 'a disease'. Something has gone awry.

Medicine has two tasks: to comfort and to heal. Yet sometimes the comforting — perhaps no more than relieving someone of a stressful environment — may itself be sufficient to alleviate illness. Disease can be literally dis*ease*. At other times, to succeed, the physician must act like a scientist. He has to diagnose a specific fault in bodily machinery and administer the corresponding drug to attack an underlying defect.

The contrast between comfort and cure is a dichotomy that can be seen throughout the history of medicine. Behind man's varied efforts to grapple with disease, from magical incantations to the intensive care of coronary victims, from attempts to thwart epidemic disease by isolation and quarantine to the psychoanalytic endeavours of Freud, Adler and Jung, there are two distinct threads. From Hippocrates onwards ill health has been interpreted as disharmony—within the body, between body and mind, between man and his environment. Or it has been seen as the result of a collision between a pathogenic (disease-carrying) agent and a susceptible individual. That agent may be internal or external; what is important is the notion of specificity, the idea that particular agents cause particular illnesses.

These twin theories have waxed and waned at different periods of history. But in the industrialised West particularly there has been an inexorable shift towards the scientific stance based on the theory known as specific aetiology. This view of disease crystallised in the seventeenth century with the work of Thomas Sydenham, and was gloriously vindicated in the nineteenth century. Louis Pasteur, Robert Koch and the other 'microbe hunters' spearheaded a triumphant series of successes in incriminating pathogenic microbes (bacteria, viruses and other microscopic forms of life) as the causes of common illnesses. Thus the mould was cast for twentieth-century medicine.

This book is an account of the strengths and weaknesses of specific aetiology. It is a personal view of the history of medicine, and my intention is to air a paradoxical truth: that the dazzling achievements of specific aetiology have now been followed by a situation where all of our major health problems—most obviously cardiovascular disease, cancers, and much mental illness—represent areas where the theory has failed. In some cases, no doubt, this is because the problems of understanding or treating those conditions are very, very difficult. Elsewhere, it seems that specific aetiology is simply the wrong tool for the job. The spectacular rewards won by the application of specific aetiology have obscured the vital importance of that twin arm of medicine: the interpretation of ill health in terms of bodily or social disharmony.

If this is so, the conclusion is not merely of academic interest. The typically Western assumption that medicine is solely or predominantly about curing illness by discrete mechanics is important politically. Whether in debates about steps towards socialised medicine in the United States, or in arguments about the allocation of resources for Britain's National Health Service, politico-economic controversy cannot be divorced from more fundamental questions of what we can and should expect of our medical practitioners. In both the privileged West and the Third World, the lessons to be learned from the increasingly apparent failures of medicine founded on the concept of specificity are not merely historical. They are economic and political.

So, while the new Indian Government in 1977 announced a plan to deal with its health problems by training a million 'barefoot doctors' rather than by investing in Western-style medicine, a debate now rages in the United States as to whether the country gets value for money out of the 150 billion dollars a year ploughed into its highly technological health system. While arguments have broken out in the medical press about the foolhardiness of immensely costly intensive care facilities for rabies victims at the All-India Institute of Medical Sciences, New Delhi, a US Senate Select Committee on Nutrition and Human Needs has identified dietary policies which they consider will make a great impact on the prevalence of heart disease, cancers, diabetes, atherosclerosis (hardening of the arteries), and cirrhosis of the liver. Even in America, it seems, there are moves to replace specific medical interventions by measures to maintain good health.

Throughout the world, the premises of traditional, prestigious, Western medicine are being challenged. Even medical research itself is experiencing a wind of change. Moving away from the notion of specific causes of disease, as documented in this book, researchers are beginning to find more meaningful clues in, for example, the geography of disease. 'Why does coronary heart disease run in families?' rather than 'What causes coronary heart disease?' is the type of question that poses itself with increasing persistence now that the conventional approach has largely failed to provide useful information about this malady. Most significant of all, one of the most exciting areas of current medical research is concerned with hereditary predisposition rather than particular agents of disease. Studies on the bodily constituents called H-LA antigens are coming very close to the Hippocratic concept of disease, which focused not on the collision between hapless victims and external, specific carriers of disease, but on bodily constitution and harmony.

In the next chapter, we shall examine the development of medicine, particularly its scientific stand, up to a point just before its greatest triumphs through the establishment of the germ theory a century ago. Chapter 3 will describe that historic breakthrough and its sequel, the proof of specific causation in other categories of illness. The remainder, and major part, of the book is intended to show that the conquests achieved by specific aetiology in recent decades are such as to have obscured from view much that is valuable in both understanding and treating ill health. While in no way minimising the potency of scientific therapies, I believe that it is both misleading and dangerous to suppose that the history of medicine is linear and that the most significant trend has been the application of scientific method to disease. Medicine is not synonymous with science.

2
Before the microbe hunters

Although scientific medicine began with the Greeks, they in turn considered the Egyptians to be the founders of the healing art. Homer, in the *Odyssey*, tells us that 'the fertile soil of Egypt is most rich in drugs, many of which are wholesome in solution, though many are poisonous'. Large numbers of potions are described in the Medical Papyri, which provide most of our knowledge of medicine in ancient Egypt. These preparations were compounded of a huge variety of ingredients, mineral, vegetable and animal. Egyptian doctors gave their drugs along with, or as part of, a spell. The gods were heavily involved in healing. Best known to us is the name of Imhotep. Almost certainly a historical person, he lived around 2700 BC and was both worshipped as a god and celebrated as a physician.

The Egyptians' demonic view of illness may well have led to the first realisation of rational therapy. Many of their drugs were foul materials, administered in the belief that they would be unwelcome to a demon possessing a patient's body. Gradually, however, cause and effect became apparent. While many of the preparations were indeed poisonous, or at least ineffective, others were potent and their effects were duly noted. In another respect too, Egyptian medicine anticipated the later, scientific stance. Practitioners specialised. There were head doctors, eye doctors, belly doctors, and others concentrating on different parts of the body. Medicine was also well organised. Doctors were paid by the state, medical treatment was available at work, and a primitive type of collective health scheme operated.

The medicine of Mesopotamia was orderly too. There were priests who specialised in diagnosis and prognosis—in reading the omens and forecasting the course of disease. There were exorcists responsible for driving out evil spirits. And physicians proper gave drugs and conducted operations. Some notion of specificity, though crude, accompanied these manoeuvres. Thus toothache was imagined to be caused by the gnawing of a worm. Babylonian physicians used about 250 plant and 120 mineral materials, as well as substances from animals. They also initiated the study of anatomy. This was a side benefit from the examination of the entrails of animals, carried out to consult the omens when people were about to embark on important ventures. Sheep's liver in particular was scrutinised closely as a guide to crucial political judgements or to the outcome of serious human illness. One Babylonian model of a sheep's liver still survives. It dates from about 2000 BC and shows the surface divided into several squares, each labelled with a different prognostication.

Hippocrates, Aristotle and Galen

Real medicine began in ancient Greece. Here the first sound knowledge was acquired of anatomy, physiology, and pathology. Here too came both the earliest realisation of external and internal causes of illness and a recognition of the broader concepts of 'constitution' or 'temperament'. Much medical nomenclature dates from the Greeks, and from three great names: Hippocrates, Aristotle, and Galen.

Hippocrates was born on the island of Cos, off the coast of Asia Minor, about 460 BC. Though we know a good deal about his ideas and method, information about the man himself is meagre. He was certainly a continual traveller, a peripatetic who practised medicine of rare quality. This he based on dedicated observation. He questioned his patients carefully, listened to them, smelt, felt and sometimes even tasted them. Hippocrates was a blend of scientist and artist. Clinical examination, he insisted, had to be rigorous. Yet it must also be based on empathy and humanity.

Underlying Hippocrates' approach was his belief in four humours: blood, yellow bile, black bile, and phlegm. The heart was supposed to be the source of blood, the brain of phlegm, the liver of yellow bile, and the spleen of black bile. Disease resulted when the humours got out of balance. Meshing conveniently with the Pythagorean idea of symmetry, the belief in four humours also became linked to Empedocles' teaching that the world consisted of four elements: fire, air, water and earth. Elements and humours were conveyors of like qualities: hot, cold, wet, and dry.

Although the terms associated with the theory (phlegmatic, humoral . . .) have passed into both general and medical usage, its basis is easily ridiculed today. What we should not overlook, however, is its positive role in directing attention towards the patient as a whole person rather than a machine, and towards the many possible determinants of ill health. Hippocrates was not interested only in symptoms and drugs; he studied nutrition too and suggested that the air, weather, and adverse temperature could be important causes of disease. The most telling phrase in his writings is 'the healing power of Nature'. Unlike so many of his predecessors, he was not over-anxious to administer medicines. Often he relied instead on 'waiting on Nature'. But this did not mean standing helplessly by. It implied good nursing, and such measures as ensuring a diet likely to aid natural recovery. Rest was the commonest stratagem required to correct an imbalance of the humours, and while any humoral excess or deficiency might be adjusted by drugs, this was considered comparatively unimportant. Hippocrates' view, and the substance of his contribution to medicine, is aptly summarised in one of his aphorisms: 'Life is short, art is long, experience is difficult.

Not only should the doctor be ready to do his duty, but the patient, the assistants, and external circumstances must conspire to effect a cure.'

Aristotle, born the son of a Macedonian physician in 384 BC, is often remembered for his erroneous notions rather than for his massive bequest to science and medicine. Such is the lot of an intellect whose monumental achievements are followed by slavish adherence to what he said, and thus the holding back of further progress. In the biological sphere, some of Aristotle's major research was in the dissection of animals (though not of the human body) and the precise descriptions of anatomy this facilitated. He *did* make mistakes (as in not distinguishing properly between arteries and veins). Yet in this work, in his primitive theory of evolution — the Ladder of Nature — and in the study of animal development, he laid the foundations for two thousand years of further research.

Following Hippocrates and Aristotle, little in the way of new ideas or observations came along in medicine until the time of Galen of Pergamon, born in AD 130. Although his fundamental attitude towards disease was not unlike that of Hippocrates (whose achievements he acknowledged continually in his own writings), his style was altogether different. Galen was a prodigious worker, a prolific writer, and an inveterate student of anatomy and physiology. Working largely if not entirely with animals, he described the arteries and veins, itemised tendons and muscles, classified bones, and introduced many terms that are still used today. Some of his most remarkable investigations were on the nervous system. From experiments on the pig's spinal cord, he found that injury between the first and second vertebrae caused instantaneous death. Cutting through the cord between the third and fourth vertebrae arrested the animal's breathing, and below the sixth vertebra it immobilised the chest muscles, leaving the diaphragm alone to maintain breathing. When he severed the cord at a lower point, the back limbs, bladder, and intestines were paralysed. These observations led him to describe in considerable detail the physiology of the spinal cord.

Arabian medicine

When Galen died, rational medicine descended into its Dark Ages. The Roman Empire was disintegrating, and those who wrote on the subject did little more than rehash earlier authors' thoughts. Only in the Arab world was there any significant activity. The tenth and eleventh centuries were the outstanding periods in the development of Islamic medicine, and two Persians, Rhazes and Avicenna, made notable progress. Both founded their studies on those of Hippocrates and Galen. Rhazes, whose *Book of the Pestilence* about smallpox is probably the first serious treatise on infectious disease, is remembered as a talented clinician and diagnostician. Among the medicines he introduced were opium-based pills for coughs, and inhalations containing sulphur for catarrh. Like the work of Rhazes, the clinical histories compiled by Avicenna are still worth reading, being based on skilled observation. He devised techniques, including a means of draining pus, which were rediscovered and applied ten centuries later. Avicenna also used an extract of wild autumn crocus (*Colchicum*) seeds to treat gout—a therapy forgotten for some nine hundred years but widely administered again today.

China—the yin and the yang

Before returning to the story of European medicine, we should examine the very different tradition of medicine in China, one that has changed probably less than any other over the centuries. The Yellow Emperor Hwang-Ti, who lived around 2700 BC, originated Chinese medicine with his work *Nei Ching*. This was devoted to internal medicine yet scarcely mentioned anatomy. The Chinese approach to health and ill health was founded on two opposing principles: the yin and the yang. The yin was a negative, female quality. The yang was active and masculine. As with the Hippocratic humours, a proper balance between the two was considered essential to health. Illness developed when the breath, the life spirit, which governed the interplay between the yin and yang, became blocked. The purpose of acupuncture, the insertion of gold or silver needles into the skin in a particular pattern, was to prevent or ameliorate such blockages.

Chinese medicine boasts few great names, because there have been few specialists. The practice of medicine has been open to all, and diet, hygiene, massage and preventive measures have long been the dominant motifs. Yet Chinese physicians have discovered genuine, effective drug treatments for disease, including mercury for syphilis and arsenic for skin conditions. In the twelfth century BC, they also pioneered a crude form of variolation, inserting material from smallpox pustules into the nostrils of healthy children in an attempt to combat epidemics.

The European anatomists

The awakening in Europe, when it occurred, was breath-taking. Better translations of Galen and Hippocrates became available and such was the inquiring spirit of the Renaissance that people were not content to learn from the work of the ancients. They began to question it. Andreas Vesalius was an outstanding questioner, and became the founder of modern anatomy and one of the chief architects of medicine as a science. His great tome *De humani corporis fabrice* ('On the structure of the human body') was published in 1543, the year in which Copernicus launched his own historic treatise showing that the Earth was not the centre of the universe. By revealing for the first time the detailed fabric of man's body, this work by Vesalius, together with that of Copernicus, shattered irretrievably the medieval speculations which had dominated thought until that time.

The son of the pharmacist to the Emperor Charles V, Vesalius was educated in Brussels and afterwards at the universities of Louvain and Paris. There he grew dissatisfied with hearing the anatomical ideas of Galen, probably based entirely on the study of non-human material, repeated uncritically, and he decided to study in Padua where dissection was being practised. He graduated in medicine there in 1537, and immediately was appointed professor of anatomy and surgery. Soon afterwards he began to compile his *Fabrica*, a seven-part treatise on different parts of the body. Systematically, Vesalius scrutinised the teachings of Galen — held in the highest esteem for a thousand years — and, by careful dissection, assembled material for his great work. As well as being the first dependable anatomical text, this also established the idea of living anatomy. For Vesalius there was no point in simply cataloguing the detailed structure of dead tissues. He was constantly interested in how the body worked. He emphasised this approach in his book and taught it to the students who flocked from all over Europe to see his demonstrations.

In 1555, in a second edition of the *Fabrica*, Vesalius went even further in challenging Galen's physiological ideas. In the first edition, for example, Vesalius conceded that, though he could not see any means of communication between the right and left ventricles (pumping chambers) of the heart, blood must nevertheless flow between the two through tiny pores — as Galen had taught. In his revised account, he said clearly that he could not accept Galen's interpretation. It was this critical temper, together with fastidious observation, which made the work of Vesalius the starting-point for the modern science of anatomy.

Science and medicine were not, of course, the only activities to be stirred into new life during the Renaissance. Some of the great artists of the time — Michelangelo, Dürer, Raphael — also started to take a close interest in the human body, and their observations conplemented those of the anatomists. Leonardo da Vinci, being a man of both art and science, also made many detailed and original investigations into the structure of man. His efforts, however, had considerably less influence at the time than those of Vesalius because he did not publish the results of his meticulous researches. Only comparatively recently have his notebooks become fully available.

Following Vesalius, a flurry of brilliant anatomists augmented man's growing knowledge of bodily machinery. Gabriello Fallopio was a pupil of Vesalius and one of his successors in the chair at Padua. His main achievement was to write about what we now know as the fallopian tubes, which carry eggs from the ovary to the uterus. He investigated the sex organs (introducing the terms 'vagina', 'clitoris' and 'placenta') and made numerous discoveries in other regions of the body, particularly the skull. He first described the space (now called the aqueduct of Fallopius) in the temporal bone through which the facial nerve passes, as well as the tympanic membrane and other structures in the ear.

Fallopio's successor was Hieronymus Fabricus. A clever anatomist and the founder of embryology, he composed the earliest account of the formation of the chick in the egg, developed an understanding of the mechanics of muscular motion, and devised a routine method for tapping fluid from the chest. But his outstanding work was his intricate description of the valves in the veins. Others had seen these before and drawn them crudely. Fabricus recorded them, in his book *De venarum ostiolis* ('On the little doors in the veins') in far greater detail than before. It was in the anatomical lecture theatre at Padua that he demonstrated the valves to his pupil William Harvey, who acquired his own interest in the circulation as a result of listening to Fabricus. Sadly, Fabricus misinterpreted the true function of the venous valves, believing that they prevented too much blood flowing away from, rather than towards, the heart. He probably made this mistake because he was still influenced by Galen's teaching.

William Harvey completes this remarkable succession of talent. By making the decisive discovery of the circulation of the blood, and the pump-like action of the heart, he originated experimental physiology. Later applied to all other regions of the body, this science became concerned not simply with describing bodily processes but also with *measuring* them.

After being educated at Cambridge and Padua, Harvey

settled in London where a meteoric career led him to become Physician Extraordinary to King James I. Harvey spent many hours each week experimenting and dissecting, and his notes show that as early as 1615 he had gained a clear insight into the circulation. He had also written of the blood passing through the lungs into the artery which leaves the left side of the heart as if driven 'by two clacks of a water-bellows to raise water'. But only after thirteen more years of careful research did he publish his classic *Exercitato anatomica de motu cordis et sanguinis* ('An anatomical treatise concerning the motion of the heart and blood').

Early in these investigations, William Harvey made two crucial finds. He realised that the venous valves allowed blood to pass only towards the heart, while those in the great arteries arising from the heart permitted blood to move only outwards into the body. The blood must therefore circulate, rather than shunt backwards and forwards in the blood vessels, as Galen had taught. It must do so continuously and always in one direction. The idea that the blood pumped through the arteries was the same blood that was collected by the veins broke entirely fresh ground.

The only missing link was the blood capillaries — the tiny vessels communicating between arteries and veins — which were revealed later by Marcello Malpighi. This discovery depended upon use of high-powered magnifying glasses which did not become available until the second half of the seventeenth century. Working chiefly at Bologna, Malpighi also broke new ground in describing the fine structure of the lung, liver, skin, spleen and kidney.

Increasingly, static anatomy was becoming dynamic anatomy, based not only on observation but also on experiments. The methods Harvey used to show that blood flows in the veins towards the heart were by cutting them, by tying ligatures to block the flow, and by observing directly the action of the valves. (Harvey dissected at least eighty species of animals.) Malpighi, too, was concerned not with dead tissues but with how things actually function. He found, for example, that the liver secretes bile through the bile duct, and that bile does not originate, as was previously supposed, in the gall bladder. So too with the work of the Dutchman Jan Swammerdam. One of his most important contributions was to disprove contemporary ideas about muscular contraction. In Swammerdam's day doctors believed that when a muscle contracted something passed into the muscle from the corresponding nerve, and thus increased its volume. By meticulously dissecting, with nerve intact, a large muscle from a frog's leg, and transferring it to a glass cylinder containing water with a sensitive capillary tube to measure changes in volume, Jan Swammerdam confirmed that this was not so. Muscles, he found, alter their shape but not their volume when they contract.

Body chemistry

Coincidentally with the development of anatomy and the forging of its link to physiology, a second strand of investigation was laying the foundations for the study of metabolism — the chemical activity characterising living cells. Santorio Sanctorius, another occupant of a chair at Padua (in medicine), is the key pioneer here. He was the first person to apply to biology and medicine the principles of exact measurement preached by his contemporary Galileo. Before being appointed at Padua, Sanctorius was physician to the King of Poland. During that time he published a book on diagnosis, which included a description of an instrument he had invented for measuring pulse rate. This was basically a simple pendulum, and the user adjusted the length of the string until the pendulum's beat coincided with the patient's pulse. As no watches then existed with second (or even minute) hands, the device was a valuable innovation. Sanctorius also introduced the clinical thermometer as a means of assessing disease.

It was after the age of fifty, however, when he went to Padua, that Sanctorius carried out his most far-reaching work, by monitoring variations in his own body weight during sleep and active movement and before and after eating and drinking. A famous woodcut shows Sanctorius sitting in his 'ballance', a chair suspended from the arm of a steelyard. Over a period of thirty years he spent as much time as possible in this device, weighing himself frequently to record changes during various physiological states. At times he even slept in the chair. He also weighed all of the food and drink he consumed, as well as his excreta. The principle aim was to measure alterations in the 'insensible perspiration' by which volatile substances were supposed to leave the body. 'That is the most proper time of Eating, wherein the Body comes to some healthful Standard, as it enjoyed the Day before, when empty,' he wrote. 'But that Apollo himself cannot find out, without the Ballance.'

Giovanni Borelli was attracted, like Sanctorius, by Galileo's advocacy of exact measurement. A mathematician by training, he treated the human body as a piece of machinery and thereby swept away the last remnants of medievalism. By analysing the mechanics of muscular movement he founded a new branch of physiology. Borelli was friendly with both Galileo and Malpighi, and became professor of mathematics at several Italian universities. His most influential work, *De motu animalium* ('On the movement of animals'), was published posthumously. In the first part, Borelli dealt with muscles and groups of muscles, interpreting their movements by geometry and mechanics as though the muscles were levers. Then he examined the process of contraction in the same way. He recognised the contractile elements in muscle, and deduced that contraction was triggered off by a 'physical reaction' travelling from the brain to the muscle via its nerve.

Animalcules in Delft

Before we turn to the implications of this wealth of discovery for theories of disease, there is one other rare achievement to recall—that of Antony van Leeuwenhoek, one of the oddest characters in the history of science. Born in Delft, Holland, in 1632, he was apprenticed at the age of sixteen to a linen draper in Amsterdam. Later he became janitor of Delft City Hall—a sinecure he held for the rest of his life and one which left him ample time to pursue his hobby of lens making. Though without formal scientific training, Leeuwenhoek was driven by insatiable curiosity to investigate the natural world. While dabbling in glass-blowing and fine metalwork, he devised a way of grinding high quality lenses and mounting them to form simple microscopes. Although these instruments were elementary in principle, Leeuwenhoek's excellent lenses and his skill with them were such that he was able to discern objects appreciably smaller than any seen with the more complex but less reliable instrument used previously.

Antony van Leeuwenhoek industriously refined his lenses and used them to scrutinise a great variety of materials — saliva, leaves, seminal fluid, urine, cow dung, circulating blood in the tail of a salamander, scrapings from his teeth, and many more. In most of his specimens he saw living creatures. Some of these we can recognise, from Leeuwenhoek's drawings, as bacteria and other microbes. Leeuwenhoek was contemptuous of many of the investigators of his day. He felt that they were too concerned with making money out of science and with boosting their personal reputations. 'But in lens grinding and discovering things hidden from our sight, these count for naught,' he wrote to the philosopher Leibniz in 1715. Although he was a secretive man, working in obscurity for forty years, Leeuwenhoek did describe the appearance of his 'animalcules' in a series of letters sent to the Royal Society in London, of which he was elected a Fellow in 1680. He would not, however, disclose the techniques employed in building his microscopes. When he died, he left behind 247 complete instruments and 172 mounted lenses, all of which he had made with his own hands. Using them, Leeuwenhoek had ended centuries of speculation about unseen forms of life.

Surprisingly, such studies were continued only sporadically over the next hundred years—probably because the lenses then generally available were so mediocre. Robert Hooke repeated Leeuwenhoek's work and gave what was probably the first demonstration in England of the microbial world, at a meeting of the Royal Society in 1677. But real progress had to await technical improvements in the microscope, which did not occur until the beginning of the nineteenth century.

The search for law and precision

Paralleling the uncovering of natural laws in the physical sciences — as disclosed by the work of Copernicus, Galileo, Kepler, and Newton — the physicians and what we would now term life scientists of the sixteenth and seventeenth centuries were applying the same methods of precise scrutiny to the human body. A mass of detail emerged, much of it buttressing an increasing conviction that the body worked like a machine. Yet this was combined with an uneasy recognition that there were as yet few rational principles, comparable with those in the physical domain, which could be applied to the practice of medicine. One attempt at such rationality came from the 'iatrophysicists' (from *iatros*, Greek for 'doctor'), who tried to explain the workings of the animal body on purely mechanical grounds. The philosopher René Descartes (see p. 118) wrote a book, published posthumously, along these lines. Descartes argued that unlike man (whose soul, he believed, resided in the pineal body the so-called 'third eye', a gland-like structure, associated with the brain, whose function is still unknown), animals had no soul and thus moved and behaved entirely automatically. The 'iatrochemists', like Jean Baptiste van Helmont, set out to interpret all life in terms of chemistry. Conversely, Georg Ernst Stahl preached the theory of vitalism — the idea that living organisms do *not* obey the laws of physics or chemistry, but operate according to principles of a wholly different kind.

'Iatrochemists and iatrophysicists gave scientific medicine quite a start,' wrote Dr Henry Sigerist in his classic *Man and*

Medicine. 'From this time on, the fate of medicine and the natural sciences is inseparably united in spite of occasional set-backs. Every natural discovery works itself out in medicine. The iatrochemists and iatrophysicists solved many problems astonishingly correctly.' Yet the influence of vitalism dates from this period too, and together the two approaches symbolise a dichotomy that has continued to the present day. That division is between those who see the body as a piece of intricate machinery which operates smoothly in health but becomes ill when in need of specific physical or chemical adjustment, and those who believe that man is not exhaustively accountable in such terms.

The search for precision did not, however, mean only the analysis of bodily structure and performance. Diseases also began to be assessed with unprecedented exactitude. Ancient medicine recognised diseased individuals, and was little concerned to differentiate distinct afflictions. That was the next major conceptual step, and it was taken by the dominating figure of clinical medicine in England in the seventeenth century, Thomas Sydenham. He made the radically new proposal that it was possible to identify specific diseases, thus distinguishing the malady from the sick person. He deduced this simply by observing that in conditions such as measles, dysentery, syphilis and gout the clinical picture was repeated unfailingly in other patients at other places and times. Sydenham was the first practitioner to diagnose measles and scarlet fever as distinct conditions and to distinguish clearly gout from rheumatism. In his classic *Methodus curandi febres* ('The method of treating fevers'), published in 1666, Sydenham suggested that some maladies were due to particular agents fighting against the natural healing powers of the body. Over three centuries later, such ideas are commonplace. In their time, they were revolutionary, and their impact far reaching.

This influence is all the more remarkable because Sydenham never taught at a university and had no students in the usual sense. Thomas Sydenham studied at Oxford, served under Cromwell in the Civil War, and in 1655 began to practise as a medical practitioner in Westminster, London. There he investigated the agues, smallpox and other fevers that were prevalent in the area. His method was a curious blend of art and science. Sydenham had little time for the microscope and the up-coming techniques of scientific analysis. He preferred instead dedicated observation at the bedside, in the style of Hippocrates, from which he built up an accurate and detailed picture of his patients' complaints. Yet Sydenham was strictly scientific about the classification of disease. Previously, physicians had rivalled the scholastic theologians in the ingenuity with which they divided and subdivided categories of malady. What they had not done was to scrutinise large numbers of cases of the conditions in questions. That was Sydenham's innovation. His compilation of thorough clinical descriptions of individual conditions was a watershed in man's understanding of disease.

For the first time, illness was seen unambiguously as a battle between the nature of man and an injury or insult. The physician's task, Sydenham believed, was to aid nature in the fight. But to do so he must understand diseases, each of which had its own peculiar characteristics. Thomas Sydenham pioneered many important practical developments, such as the use of quinine for malaria, laudanum to relieve pain, and iron preparations to treat blood disorders. But his major achievement—and a step which, once taken, could not be reversed— was in placing the concept of specificity in the centre of physicians' minds. As a tool, this had profound repercussions in both medical practice and medical research.

One immediate result of Sydenham's efforts was a spate of books containing really accurate descriptions of distinct diseases. By the end of the century, many excellent monographs existed on tuberculosis, rickets, and other conditions. Attention also turned to occupational ill health, and an Italian doctor, Bernadino Ramazzini, wrote his classic *De morbis artificium diatriba* ('A treatise on the diseases of tradesmen'), which dealt with illnesses associated with forty different trades.

Then came Carl Linnaeus, a physician turned naturalist who devoted his life to classifying, recording, and naming living creatures. Linnaeus introduced the binominal system for itemising scientifically different genera and species of plants and animals, each being given a two-part name consisting of genus and species. Using this method, he published his great compilation, *Systema naturae*, in 1735. So why not regiment maladies on a similar basis? One man who tried to do so was Linnaeus's contemporary, Boissier de Sauvages, who was also both a physician and a botanist. In the mid-eighteenth century he published a disease system constructed in this way, 'written in the spirit of Sydenham and according to botanists' methods'. This in turn influenced Linnaeus, who produced his own version. Nosology, the systematisation of diseases according to their symptoms, became a popular occupation.

Some good came of this. More infections that had been confused previously, such as typhus, typhoid fever, and malaria, were distinguished correctly. But grandiose attempts to order all diseases like birds or flowers—the most ambitious being Philippe Pinel's classification of over 2,500 afflictions into species, orders, and families—failed and were forgotten.

What we do owe to this period is an increasingly clear picture of specific, constant, repeatable illness as opposed to a more vague view of ill health. This did not emerge without heated debate. Much of it devolved upon developments in pathological anatomy, principally in Paris at the turn of the century. A key figure, though not a man of great influence in his time, was René Laennec, best known today as the inventor of the stethoscope. He did rather more than that. Laennec applied rare skill in exploring the physical signs in the chest which provide clues to a wide range of different diseases. Present day methods and the terminology of chest examination owe a great deal to him.

According to Sir William Osler, in *The Evolution of Modern Medicine*, publication in 1819 of Laennec's book on auscultation (listening to body sounds as an aid to diagnosis, usually with the stethoscope) marked the beginning of a new era in medicine: 'The clinical recognition of individual diseases had made really very little progress; with the stethoscope begins the day of physical diagnosis. The clinical pathology of the heart, lungs and abdomen was revolutionised, Laennec's book is in the category of the eight or ten greatest contributions to the science of medicine.'

But Laennec was a poor lecturer, and a far more influential figure in the Paris School was the colourful Breton, François Broussais. Paradoxically, though his work spawned more evidence of specific causes of disease, he himself appeared to resist this conclusion. Broussais worked hard to stimulate the study of morbid anatomy, from which he showed that some afflictions produced distinctive changes in the tissues. He interpreted what he saw, however, as the reactions of the body to different degrees of irritation. This was then strongly disputed by the work of Pierre Bretonneau who, on the basis of intensive studies of diphtheria and typhoid fever, stressed that the important distinction between pathological appearances was their essential nature rather than their intensity. The debates of the morbid anatomists had had another beneficial effect — they had added to the nosologists' preoccupation with symptoms a further consideration, disease as a cause of changes in *function*.

As the eighteenth century opened, Richard Mead, physician to Queen Anne, had this to say about the importance of mathematics in relation to medicine:

Since of late mathematicians have set themselves to the study of it [medicine] men do already begin to talk so intelligibly and comprehensibly even about abstruse matters that it may be hoped in a short time that those who are designed for this profession are early, while their minds and bodies are patient of labour and toil, initiated in the knowledge of numbers and geometry, that mathematical learning will be the distinguishing mark of a physician from a quack; and that he who wants this necessary qualification will be as ridiculous as one without Greek or Latin.

Nearly two centuries later, in a presidential address to the British Medical Association in 1888, Sir William Gardner said:

> . . . most of the great advances in medical diagnosis in the present day, through the stethoscope, microscope, laryngoscope, ophthalmoscope, sphymograph, electricity as applied to muscle and nerve, etc, involve applications of pure physics which are neither remote from practice nor yet very easily mastered by the beginner; [since] in the case of electricity and other physical reagents, even heat and cold, etc., we are every day extending the domain of these sciences in therapeutics, and still more perhaps in preventive medicine and sanitary science, their claim for an extended recognition in teaching seems enormously enhanced. I am persuaded that in a very few years the physical laboratory will become an absolutely essential preliminary step in the education of the physician. of the future, and that those who have not undergone this training will be hopelessly distanced in the race.

The period between these significantly similar statements saw a steady acceleration in the application of physics, chemistry and mathematics to the human body. It was not merely that these disciplines generated gadgets which could aid the physician. The new disclosures encouraged medical men to think of the body, and its battles with disease, in specific, mechanistic terms. At a time when doctors were still largely impotent to deal with serious maladies, the promise afforded by the burgeoning discoveries of natural science was understandably influential.

The contribution of science

Stephen Hales was a polymath whose work typifies the new marriage between medicine and science. Although a clergyman by training, he did historic research in human physiology, chemistry, and plant physiology. His interests in all three fields were united around the similarity he perceived between respiration in animals and the process of combustion. Hales was also one of the first experimenters to emphasise the vital necessity of quantitative measurement in physiological and chemical experiments. After studying at Cambridge he became Perpetual Curate of Teddington in 1709. He refused preferment several times, on the grounds that it would interfere with his scientific studies in his country parsonage.

Perhaps the greatest innovation of Hales was to measure blood pressure. He achieved this by inserting tubes into the arteries and veins of various animals and observing both the height to which the blood rose and its variations with the heartbeat. This was a breakthrough of potentially great clinical importance. For Hales it was part of a rigorous scientific investigation of the circulatory system, during which he calculated circulation rate and estimated the velocity of blood in the arteries, veins, and capillaries.

A versatile contemporary of Hales, Albrecht von Haller, was the man whose *Elementa physiologiae corporis humani* ('The elements of the physiology of the human body') launched the modern phase of this science, by summarising critically the whole of the physiological knowledge of his day. As well as being a physiologist, Haller was a distinguished poet, novelist, botanist and anatomist. Born in Berne, Switzerland, he worked both there and in Göttingen. Several of Haller's discoveries are of historic permanence — he was, for example, the first person to describe respiration adequately. But his greater significance was in modernising man's conceptual picture of the working of the human body and nervous control in particular.

Haller began by examining muscle fibres, in which he recognised what he termed irritability — the capacity to contract in response to a minutely small stimulus and then return to their former length. (He saw this quality not only in the muscles of limbs but also in the heart and intestines.) Haller thus distinguished between 'inherent muscular force' and 'nerve force'. Next he considered the process of feeling, showing that the tissues themselves were not capable of sensation, which depended rather upon the nerves. He also demonstrated that all nerves are centred towards the brain. From this and related research, Haller began to sketch a map of nervous regulation as we now recognise it, with the brain and central nervous system as the co-ordinating unit for impulses flowing outwards and inwards through different nerves. Albrecht von Haller was conspicuously rational. He rejected mystical ideas and all of his work was firmly grounded in experiment rather than armchair speculation.

Of all the departments of the body, the nervous system was the last to succumb to scientific exploration. Compared with muscles, analysed in terms of forces and levers, or the circulation, traced like a plumbing system, nerves are considerably more intractable to investigation. Following Haller, the two men who took inquiry a stage further were a German, Johannes Müller, and a Pole, Robert Remak. Working in Berlin, Müller was the author of the 'law of specific nervous energies'. This states that each sensory nerve, however stimulated, gives rise to its own particular sensation and no other. Conversely, the same stimulus offered to different sense organs results in a characteristic sensation in each organ. Thus any type of stimulation, whether thermal, electrical, or mechanical, produces a sensation of light when applied to the optic nerve. The auditory, olfactory and other nerves also respond in their own distinctive way whatever the nature of the stimulus. As well as describing the operation of a further area of bodily machinery, Müller's law has philosophical implications: external reality may not be as real as we suppose. Müller also broke new ground in linking his interest in the nervous system with human behaviour. One of his aphorisms was: 'No one can be a psychologist without being a physiologist.'

Robert Remak, who was born in Poland but worked in Berlin, initially with Müller, was largely responsible for initiating the microscopic scrutiny of the body's nerve network. In his doctoral thesis, he reported his finding that the inner 'axons' of nerves in the central nervous system were sheathed in a material called myelin. (Later in the same year Theodor Schwann described myelin sheaths independently and his name, rather than Remak's, has since become associated with the discovery.) Remak also showed that the nerve fibres of the sympathetic nervous system (that which does not respond to conscious control) are grey, rather than white, because they do not have myelin sheaths. Thirdly, he discerned that the axons of nerves throughout the body arose from cells in the spinal cord, running continuously from there to their terminal branchings. Many other discoveries followed, including his recognition of six distinct layers in the cerebral cortex (the outer 'grey matter' of the brain). His researches also led him into a significant new field — that of electroconvulsive therapy, used today to treat severe depression and related conditions. ECT owes its origin to Remak, who wrote the first serious book on the subject in 1858.

With this work by Robert Remak, we arrive at the modern phase of medical science. The climate was now becoming highly favourable for the reception of the theory of specific aetiology, which we shall be considering in the next chapter. The period is symbolised by the work of Claude Bernard. He was the founder of experimental medicine — the artificial production, by chemical and physical stratagems, of disease and conditions mimicking disease. This is now widely and successfully used as a method of investigating how the body performs in normal health, and how ill health disrupts one or other of its functions.

Claude Bernard was educated at the Jesuit College in Ville-franche, the town of his birth, and at Thoissey. After working as a pharmacist in Lyons, he went to Paris to enter the School of Medicine there. He graduated as a doctor of medicine in 1853 and began his distinguished career in physiology. In 1854 he became the first occupant of the chair of experimental physiology at the Sorbonne, where he did his great work in experimental medicine. The worlds of science and medicine plied him with honours in recognition of many historic achievements and in 1869 he was declared a Senator of the French Empire by imperial decree.

One of Bernard's most important findings was that the liver stores glucose in the form of glycogen. First he showed that when a dog was fed a diet containing sugar, glucose appeared in the portal vein, which leads from the gut to the liver, and in the hepatic veins connecting the liver to the general circulation. In an animal given a protein diet without sugar there was no glucose in the portal vein, but a high concentration in the hepatic veins. Then in 1857 Bernard found that the liver maintained a store of glucose as glycogen, and released it when needed. Until that time, it was thought that only plants could build up complex chemicals as well as break them down. This was the beginning of our knowledge of carbohydrate metabolism, which has had practical consequences in the treatment of diabetes and glycogen-storage diseases, where the system observed by Bernard goes awry.

Bernard realised that pancreatic juice was involved in digesting fats in food. This he deduced by observing the action of the juice on fat in a test tube and by noting the appearance of a white fluid in the rabbit gut, but only below the point at which the pancreatic duct entered the duodenum. He found too that pancreatic juice broke down starch into the sugar maltose. This provided the first clues to the digestive function of the pancreas, which had been thought of previously as a salivary gland.

The control of blood flow by the nervous system was one of Bernard's other major discoveries. In 1815, he cut the cervical sympathetic nerve in a rabbit and noticed that that side of the animal's head became warmer. This was due to relaxation of constriction of the tiny blood capillaries; stimulating the cut end of the nerve made them contract. Later he learned that the nervous system contained separate fibres which had the opposite effect—they made the blood capillaries dilate.

Claude Bernard was interested in the action of poisons because he realised he could gain information about the body from the ill effects they caused. By studying the effect of carbon monoxide, for example, he found that oxygen is not simply dissolved in the blood but is carried from the lungs to the tissues of the body by the red blood corpuscles. In 1857 he demonstrated that injection of curare, the South American arrow-poison, poisons the endings of the nerves in muscles throughout the body. Afterwards, a muscle can no longer be stimulated through its nerve, but will still react to a direct stimulus. This work led eventually to the modern use of curare, alongside anaesthetics, to relax patients' muscles during certain operations.

Despite this string of experimental breakthroughs, Claude Bernard himself did not favour a simplistic, mechanical interpretation of living processes. Indeed, he introduced the concept of the *milieu intérieur*, meaning the constancy of the internal chemistry of the body and the co-ordinated regulation of its various parts. This delicate and complex balance was essential to health. Alas, many of those who have followed Bernard have been more impressed by his experimental techniques than by his overall philosophy. Numerous failures and errors can be attributed to a neglect of his wider message.

The mystery of epidemics

There is one more antecedent to the theory of specific aetiology: the growing suspicion that epidemic disease might be spread by some form of contagion. Another modern commonplace, it is difficult today for us to understand why the real nature of infection took so long to be recognised. Just as puzzling is why the belief in communicable disease, when it did begin to take light, was usually held much more strongly by the common people than by the medical profession.

After all, the possibility that plagues were transmitted by contagion had long been implied by the occurrence of epidemics, probably since Neolithic man first gathered himself into village communities. However, the mechanism of such contagion was long obscure. In the *Iliad*, Homer describes how

Apollo caused epidemic disease in the Achaean army besieging Troy, and the motion of divine judgement through pestilence was a compelling one for early man. Gradually, however, this theurgical theory became supplanted by more natural explanations such as 'noxious miasms', the influence of the seasons, 'bad air' and, later, 'electrical forces'.

Greek medicine reached no conclusions about the basis of contagion. But the Bible helped. Several passages teach that he who touches one who is 'unclean' becomes defiled himself. Those suffering from leprosy are considered particularly unclean, and Leviticus (13 and 14) gives detailed instructions for dealing with this disease, including isolation of the sick and the disinfection of their clothes and belongings. The Christian church set out to enforce these rules and began a war against leprosy. In the Middle Ages public health measures, stemming from the biblical treatment of the leper, were used to limit the spread of a series of great epidemics. Segregation imposed during the Black Death of 1347 - 8 and the plague in Milan and Venice between 1370 and 1374 was seen to be most effective when most severe. Smallpox and typhus outbreaks, the mysterious 'English sweats' (probably a severe virus infection) from 1485 to 1551, and a pandemic of syphilis during the sixteenth century all confirmed that disease could be communicated rapidly throughout a community after being introduced by one ill person. Containment was frequently enforced when the nature of the affliction was hazy or unknown.

Indeed, what is remarkable about the successes of such measures is that they were used with little or no understanding of the nature of the enemy. The Jewish people in particular, though they did not contribute significantly to curative medicine, developed a sanitary system that was highly effective. The American sanitation specialist Dr Thurman Rice in his book *The Conquest of Disease* insists that: 'Moses must be classed as one of the world's greatest sanitarians. It was no small task to take a great horde of the Israelites into a desert and keep them well for a period of 40 years. It is astonishing that they were not decimated annually by all manner of filth and parasitic disease such as afflicted our troops in the Civil and Spanish-American wars.' The main reason why the Jewish people escaped the ravages of epidemic infection is probably to be found in Deuteronomy (23), which lays down explicit instructions for disposing of human wastes. Moses also devised elaborate rules for the division of things into clean and unclean. Meat inspection was rated as highly important. While some of these practices were largely ceremonial, most were in some way related to the preservation of life.

Another empirical measure introduced to staunch the proliferation of disease was quarantine. The word owes its origin to attempts to keep bubonic plague out of the Republic of Ragusa, on the eastern side of the Adriatic, in the late fourteenth century. The infection was then spreading through Europe, but Venice had contrived to remain free of it by way of regulations ensuring that people must wait outside the city for a specified period before entering. The Ragusa authorities set up a landing-stage far from the city and harbour, where intending visitors suspected of carrying the disease had to spend thirty days in the open air and sunlight. This interval, known as the *trentina*, proved to be too short. So it was extended to forty days, the *quarantina*. Together with the incineration of all goods belonging to people found to be afflicted, quarantine became routine in many parts of Europe. During the eighteenth century, drastically enforced in France during a bubonic plague epidemic in Marseilles, it was clearly effective in containing the infection. Quarantine is one of very few medical or sanitary advances we owe to the Middle Ages.

From Hippocrates to Darwin

Epidemic disease gives us the most vivid illustration of the changed approach between the time of Hippocrates and the mid-nineteenth century. In the first book of his *Epidemics*, Hippocrates reports an outbreak on the Island of Thasos:

There resulted many cases of burning fever of a quite benign nature. Nose bleeding was an occasional symptom. There were no deaths among these cases. Many had swellings near the ear, some unilateral, and some bilateral. Most of the patients were without fever and not confined to bed. There were some who had mild fever. The swellings disappeared without scars and none became infected, as is usually the case with swellings originating from other causes. The swellings were large, soft, extensive without inflammation and pain. They vanished without a trace. They occurred in boys, youths and adult muscular men especially in those who visited the gymnasia and arenas. Few women were taken ill. Many of those who were sick had coughs without expectoration and their voices were hoarse. After a longer or shorter period there appeared painful enlargements of the testicles, sometimes unilateral, sometimes bilateral, some had fever and some not. Most of these complained much.

Two features of this passage are striking. First, Hippocrates wrote a clear and accurate description, perfectly acceptable by modern standards, of mumps. Second, he gave the disease no name. We now know it as parotitis epidemica — an epidemic inflammation of the parotid (salivary) gland. Much medical history since the time of Hippocrates — much of it based on less acute observation — has been concerned to differentiate and specify discrete diseases. Yet the Greek master himself leaves us a superb portrait of the condition, without any inclination to label it with a precise designation.

The reason for this omission is that Hippocratic medicine focused not on diseases but on man himself. It recognised sick people, in all their human variability, rather than distinct maladies. One can pick out the beginnings of disease concepts in antiquity, but somehow they never matured. Hippocratic medicine was concerned above all with constitution. Every one of us, Hippocrates taught, has an individual temperament, so treatment for illness must always be individual. Fat, thin, energetic, docile, rich or poor, we all react differently to stimuli and to changes in our circumstances, including illness. So what determines the course of a disease is not its nature but the type of person who is afflicted. The theory of humours also provided a theoretical basis for the notion that in each human being one of the four humours predominates, and thus influences that person's character.

There is much truth in the Hippocratic recognition of constitution, but it is a truth that was eclipsed by the inexorable drive of scientific inquiry. As we have seen in this chapter, first the anatomists, then the physiologists, chemists and physicists began to assemble a very different picture of man. What they discovered, time and time again, was that the human body is built to a common plan, like a machine off a production line. One fibula, one pharynx or cardinal ligament looks like, and functions like, any other. The body is wonderfully constructed, but it is rational and understandable and—despite appearances—one model is the same as the next.

Science thrives on regularity, on discerning pattern and sameness in material and phenomena, so as it shook off humoral speculations and mysticism, it surged ahead. And when we reach the nineteenth century science was in its heyday of determinism. The eighteenth century was a time of order in science—typified by the achievements of Linnaeus—and of attempts in geology, biology and other disciplines to attain mathematical precision and finality. Most of these efforts were premature. But a hundred years later, with the work of Dalton, Davy, Faraday, Clerk Maxwell and others, order seemed to prevail. Cause and effect became the guiding principle for Victorian scientists.

In the mid-nineteenth century, too, Charles Darwin incubated and eventually published his theory of evolution. Founded on over twenty years' work, beginning with his observations in the Galapagos Islands during a voyage of the *Beagle*, the theory shattered the beliefs of the religious (though Darwin said he had no wish to do so), provided ammunition for economic determinism, and above all established a rational framework for understanding the development and nature of life on earth. Not only were the black man, the white man, and the yellow man of the same stock; *Homo sapiens* was also part of the animal world. Darwin confirmed for all time the unity of the rich variety of life on earth.

Such was the mood of the times into which the doctrine of specific aetiology, in all its stark clarity, was born. But the moment does not necessarily bring forth the man. As we shall see in the next chapter, a favourable climate and mere competence were not enough. Acceptance of specific aetiology — despite the forces running in its favour — depended upon near-genius allied to a pedantic insistence on the highest standards of proof. There was a measure of good fortune too.

3
Magic bullets

On 5 May 1881, a large crowd gathered on a farm at Pouilly-le-Fort in France to watch the first part of a historic demonstration. Louis Pasteur with two assistants, Charles Chamberland and Emile Roux, and a flock of sheep held the centre of the stage. The purpose of the exercise was to see whether sheep could be protected against a ghastly and usually deadly disease: anthrax. Pasteur had been claiming as much, and his boasts had met disbelieving ridicule.

With his jaunty limp, Pasteur walked into the arena like a matador and bowed to the assembled throng — a mixed assembly of Senators of the Republic, scientists, horse doctors and farmers. His colleagues carried syringes and flasks containing the preparation which they believed would immunise the animals against anthrax. They went together to the sheds where the sheep were divided into two groups. Then they injected the supposed vaccine into the thighs of twenty-four of the animals, which were labelled by a little gouge punched out of their ears. An equal number of sheep were left without injections. Next, everyone repaired to a large hall on the farm, where Pasteur lectured for half an hour, explaining simply and logically what he had done and what he expected to follow.

Twelve days later, there was a repeat performance. The crowd assembled again and Pasteur and his team injected vaccine, a 'stronger' type this time, into the same batch of sheep. He was confident of the outcome of the experiment, perhaps uncertain only whether he would be *totally* vindicated. 'If the success is complete', he wrote to his son-in-law, 'this will be one of the finest examples of applied science in this century, consecrating one of the greatest and most fruitful discoveries.'

On 31 May the most dangerous part of the drama was enacted. Before another huge body of spectators, Émile Roux administered a fatal dose of virulent anthrax bacilli to all forty-eight sheep—both vaccinated and unvaccinated. One sceptic insisted that he use a larger quantity than intended, and a fastidious veterinary surgeon demanded that the lethal organisms should be given alternatively to sheep from the two groups. Pasteur was happy to comply. By 3.30 p.m., the task was complete, and everyone agreed to return on 2 June to see the result.

The audience which converged on the farm on the appointed day was even larger than those earlier. This time there were General Councillors as well as Senators; delegates from the Agricultural Society of Melun, the Central Council of Hygiene of Seine et Marne, and various medical and veterinary societies; as well as many farmers and inquisitive spectators who had been reading a mixture of dismissive and optimistic articles about the tests in their newspapers.

When Pasteur and his assistants walked onto the field at 2 p.m., they met mighty applause. The carcases of twenty-two of the twenty-four unvaccinated sheep lay on the grass, and the two survivors were in the last throes of anthrax, with black blood oozing from their mouths and noses. Every one of the vaccinated sheep was in perfect health.

Louis Pasteur was fond of public demonstrations to prove scientific points and this was his most sensational to date. Three days later, one of his former critics, a M. Bouley, who was General Inspector of Veterinary Schools, wrote to him:

Dearest Master, your triumph has filled me with joy. Though the days are long past now when my faith in you was still somewhat hesitating, not having sufficiently impregnated my mind with your spirit, as long as the event—which has just been realised in a manner so rigorously in conformity with your predictions — was still in the future, I could not keep myself from feeling a certain anxiety... The world has found you faithful to all your promises, and you have enscribed one more great date in the annals of science, and particularly those of medicine, for which you have opened a new era.

The incredibly exact outcome of the Pouilly-le-Fort exercise illustrates the power of the notion of specific aetiology. What Pasteur had done was to take the particular germ responsible for anthrax, to weaken it so that it was no longer able to cause disease but *was* still capable of protecting an animal against that disease, and then to prove its efficacy against the microbe in its most virulent form. The mathematically precise result underlined the potency of the ideas behind the demonstration. Pasteur's vaccine would have been totally ineffective against any other microorganism except the anthrax bacillus. The basis of his experiment — and the source of his confidence — was the one-to-one relationship between a disease and its specific causative agent.

The origin of organisms

As we saw in Chapter 2, conditions were particularly favourable in the mid-nineteenth century for the acceptance of such a notion. Thomas Sydenham and others had explored the concept of specificity, and the steady advance of materialistic medicine had rendered the ground even more fertile. When specific aetiology did arrive, it came part and parcel with the germ theory. But this could not flourish until one other idea had been cleared away: that of spontaneous generation.

Both medieval and Renaissance scientific writers thought that living creatures could arise spontaneously. It was a reasonable belief. Judges (14) records the sudden appearance of a swarm of bees in a lion carcass, and in the scientific world spontaneous generation (heterogenesis) had been authenticated by Aristotle. The idea was scarcely questioned until 1688, when the Italian physician Francesco Redi showed that maggots did not develop in decaying meat when he used gauze to protect it from contamination by flies. He went on to trace the metamorphosis of eggs, through maggots, into flies of various sorts. Redi was a true scientist with an inquiring mind who wrote of once having believed things 'which I am now ashamed to remember'. His demonstration, and ample confirmation by other experimenters, soon effectively discredited belief in the spontaneous generation of visible organisms such as maggots, grubs, flies, and bees.

After the discovery of microscopic life towards the end of the seventeenth century, however, such an origin still seemed more than plausible for the tiny 'animalcules' found in infusions* of hay and other organic materials. Discussion of the spontaneous origin of these creatures afforded more protracted controversy. In 1799, the Italian Abbé Lazzaro Spallanzini found he could prevent animalcules from appearing in infusions by boiling the extracts for at least forty minutes. The Englishman John Needham, who was both a scientist and a Catholic divine, objected that the heat destroyed a necessary 'vegetative force' in the air. But this was later answered by other experimenters—most convincingly in 1854 by Heinrich Schröder and Theodor von Dusch. They showed that air which was unheated but filtered through cotton wool did not necessarily cause the development of animalcules in infusions.

At about this time, the French naturalist Félix-Archimède Pouchet was loudly claiming experimental verification of heterogenesis, and this led Louis Pasteur to take an interest in the problem. He commenced a long series of exhaustive and well controlled experiments, in which he showed that living creatures did not appear in sterilised food materials unless such creatures were introduced from outside. Later published in a classic paper in 1861, this work provided a convincing indictment of spontaneous generation. After renewed boasts

*Hence the origin of the term 'infusoria'.

by Pouchet, Pasteur also mounted a public demonstration, at the Sorbonne on 7 April 1864, which remained unanswered by his opponent. Some of Pasteur's sealed flasks of nutrient broth remain to this day—with no sign of incipient life. After the Sorbonne display, belief in heterogenesis quickly died away. Its demise was greatly assisted in Britain by the lectures, articles and tireless demonstrations of John Tyndall (who also proved that some bacteria can become spores, which are ultra-resistant to heat). Clear refutation of this Aristotelean belief was an essential preliminary to the acceptance of the germ theory of disease.

Exploring the microbial world

Another precursor of specific aetiology was increasing curiosity about the microbial world. After the hiatus following the work of Antony von Leeuwenhoek, technical improvements in the microscope at the beginning of the nineteenth century stimulated fresh interest in life invisible to the naked eye. One result was a tome on the infusoria, published in 1838 and written by Christian Ehrenberg. Ferdinand Cohn studied under Ehrenberg in Berlin and later became one of the pioneers of systematic bacteriology, classifying bacteria by their shape and physiology. Several scientists at that time, notably Ernst Hallier, were influenced by the discovery of variations in shape and form (pleomorphism) in fungi. They came to believe that bacteria too were extremely variable organisms, being either innumerable different forms of a universal 'panbacillus' or stages in the development of fungi. Cohn and his school, working in Breslau, Silesia, rejected these claims and argued that individual species of bacteria behave predictably when grown in a particular way, and may therefore be identified and classified. This view proved to be essentially correct. It was a vital prerequisite to the theory of specific aetiology (though was not established unambiguously until late in the nineteenth century).

Probably the first scientific report of disease caused by a transmissible parasitic microorganism was by Agostino Bassi in his book *Del mal del segno*, published in 1835. Bassi was an Italian lawyer and part time scientist. In his book he described the organism responsible for the fatal and thus economically disastrous muscardine disease of the silkworm, and its transmission by contact or by infected food. Bassi suggested that the condition was disseminated via 'seeds' produced by the fungus. Despite the historic nature of this work (the fungus was later named *Botrytis bassiana* in honour of its discoverer), and an enthusiastic reception by botanists and agriculturalists, it did not impress the physicians. The one exception was Johann Schönlein. Introducing his own identification, in 1839, of the fungus (now called *Achorion schönleinii*) responsible for the form of ringworm known as favus, he wrote: 'You are familiar, without doubt, with Bassi's beautiful discovery of the nature of *muscardine*. The fact seems to me of the greatest interest for pathology, although to my knowledge not a single physician up to this time has found it worthy of his attention.'

Chemistry and life

That doctors neglected a piece of work with such revolutionary implications is significant. When the great breakthrough came, it was not through medicine but through science and a scientist: Louis Pasteur. The route was via the age-old phenomena of fermentation and putrefaction. Fermentation, harnessed in making wine, beer, and bread, must have been one of the first biological processes which man adapted for his own domestic purposes. However, yeast was shown to be a living organism only in 1837, independently by Theodor Schwann, Friedrich Kützing and Charles Caignard-Latour. From the fact that yeast invariably occurred in fermenting material, and that the activity ceased when the yeast was destroyed, Schwann concluded that the living organisms actually caused the fermentation. As so often happens in science, other investigators were unable to reproduce this experiment with the same results and it was largely forgotten until Pasteur took up the subject some twenty years later.

Meanwhile, chemistry had been developing confidently and chemists were beginning to examine living material. In 1789 Antoine Lavoisier had found that he could express quantitatively the conversion of sugar into alcohol and carbon dioxide in vinous fermentation; the same quantities of end products always came from the same amount of starting material. Then in 1828 in Berlin Friedrich Wöhler synthesised an organic substance, previously thought to be formed only by living cells, from simple inorganic materials. This was urea, a substance we excrete as a result of digesting protein. These findings led to increasing support for the theory, trumpeted by Wöhler and Justus von Liebig, that fermentation was essentially a chemical phenomenon. A battle then raged between their view and that of Caignard-Latour, Schwann, and Kützing, who believed that fermentation was inseparable from living organisms. There was something 'vital' about the process which could not be reduced to mere chemistry. The ensuing dispute, which became confused with the controversy over spontaneous generation, was doubly unfortunate because the antagonists were both partly correct. Whilst the biological theory was the immediate victor, the chemical interpretation proved to be sound too, at the turn of the century, when enzymes — the catalytic proteins responsible for metabolism — were first isolated from living cells.

Louis Pasteur was born the son of a tanner on 27 December 1822. He studied at the École Normale Supérieure in Paris, where he fell under the influence of the great chemist André Dumas — and resolved that he too should be a great chemist. He became fascinated by crystallography, and for his doctorate he did pioneering work in the field now known as stereochemistry. At the age of twenty-six, peering at crystals of tartaric acid and its salts, he discovered that some compounds previously thought to be uniform in composition had more than one crystal form, often mirror images of each other. In addition to demonstrating that such 'optical isomers' existed, he devised ways of isolating them from the mixtures in which they usually occur. One method was to separate the crystals painstakingly by hand, under a magnifying lens. The other made use of fungi that consumed one isomer but not the other. In this way, Louis Pasteur became impressed by the precision of microbes, which can distinguish chemicals that are in every way identical save for tiny differences in the orientation of the facets on their crystals.

In 1854 Pasteur was appointed Professor of Chemistry and Dean of Sciences in the University of Lille. Fermentation industries were important in that city, and one of the manufacturers, a M. Bigo, suggested that Pasteur might interest himself in some of their problems. Why, for example, did vinegar sometimes turn sour during its production from beet juice? What made wine and beer manufacture 'go wrong' occasionally, when the same, traditional routines were followed impeccably year by year? Pasteur first tackled the souring of milk, a process accompanied by the formation of lactic acid. He published his findings in 1857. In that paper, Pasteur proved that microorganisms caused the souring, though he was not able to separate them from the milk. He then went on to investigate the alcoholic fermentation of wine and beer, the formation of acetic acid to make vinegar, and the appearance of butyric acid when butter goes rancid. After a period spent studying the *pébrine* disease that was then devastating the French silk industry, Pasteur resumed these investigations six years later. His classic *Études sur la bière* describing the results appeared in 1871.

Pasteur concluded that the various biochemical activities — production of alcohol, lactic, butyric and acetic acids — were brought about by corresponding, specific microorganisms. He was helped to this verdict by the results observed when his relatively crude cultures became contaminated. Thus experiments on the souring of milk almost always finished with the same microbes in the curd — different microbes from those found in other fermentations. But sometimes tests gave an

anomalous result. On occasions, sour milk yielded butyric acid
instead of lactic acid. When this happened, Pasteur found that
a different organism — the one usually responsible for causing
rancidity in butter — was invariably present.

Fermentation and disease

With a constant interest in the practical relevance of science,
Pasteur then applied his work to various 'diseases' affecting the
wine industry at the time. To the amazement of the vintners,
he was soon able to diagnose conditions such as 'ropy wine',
'oily wine', and 'bitter wine', simply by examining a drop
under the microscope and seeing what microbes the wine contained.

The similarity between putrefaction of dead animal or plant
material and suppuration, particularly in war wounds, was
underlined in the nineteenth century by studies of septic complications in surgical wounds. The arrival of anaesthesia had
been a mixed blessing. In the middle of the century, Thomas
Morton in Boston and James Simpson in Edinburgh had
pioneered the successful use of ether during surgical operations. Others were taking up their lead. But by facilitating
surgery these advances inevitably made more conspicuous the
frequently harrowing consequence of vile, suppurating
wounds. Caignard-Latour and Schwann first discovered the
microbial basis of putridity in 1837, and in 1863 Pasteur
proved that suppuration was caused by 'organised ferments' —
microorganisms.

Following Louis Pasteur's key discovery, Joseph Lister
worked on wound suppuration in Glasgow during the 1860s
and introduced antiseptic surgery using a spray of carbolic
acid playing over the operation site. In 1877 Lister read to the
Pathological Society his paper entitled 'On the lactic fermentation and its bearing on Pathology'. With further experiments
to support the earlier researches of Pasteur, Lister tried to
convince his colleagues that growth of specific microorganisms

was responsible for specific fermentative changes. By implication, a similar relationship might obtain in surgical wounds.

Meanwhile, Pasteur was beginning to apply to a series of human and animal diseases—including anthrax, chicken cholera, swine erysipelas and rabies—the lessons he had learned from studies of fermentation. From 1877 until he died in 1895, he investigated each condition with two objectives: to isolate and cultivate the organism responsible and to devise methods of controlling the infection. In 1879, he had a piece of luck. He found that chickens injected with an old culture of chicken cholera bacilli did not develop the disease. And a fresh preparation, capable of killing chickens, was harmless when administered to those chicks that had already received the old culture. Pasteur thus learned the trick of 'attenuation', a weakening of the virulence of microorganisms by ageing (or other methods), without any alteration in their capacity to confer resistance. This became the basis for several vaccines and was the technique used on the farm at Pouilly-le-Fort.

No doubt Pasteur was helped in making this discovery by the empirical knowledge of immunity that already existed. It had long been apparent that recovery from many diseases was followed by a period—perhaps a lifetime—of invulnerability to further attacks. Also, the use of an aged culture was an accident, not a calculated tactic. But it would be totally wrong to explain the incident in these terms alone. The great French chemist's life work included far too many 'lucky' accidents for that to be an acceptable description. Perhaps the most apposite comment is Pasteur's own aphorism: 'chance favours the prepared mind'.

Meanwhile too, the importance of Ferdinand Cohn's criticism of pleomorphism was looming large. Cohn was a dedicated individual, who has been virtually eclipsed in accounts of the development of bacteriology by the more flamboyant pioneers. He is not mentioned, for example, in Paul de Kruif's book *Microbe Hunters*, which contains vivid pen portraits of the other great names. The reason for this neglect is twofold. Cohn was a scientist in a field dominated in its early days by medical men. But he lacked the showmanship of Pasteur, with his sensational public demonstrations, and he worked in a discipline which at first glance appears infinitely dull. He regimented organisms into tidy groups.

Cohn's principal achievement, an account of which appeared in print in 1872, was to show that bacteria can be classified, like plants and animals, as species and genera. Thus, he established, in his *Untersuchungen über Bacterien*, that rod-like bacilli do not transmute capriciously into spherical cocci, or vice versa. Species are fixed and unchanging. The experiments he conducted to confirm these facts occupied many years of intensive research at Breslau, where he was a professor of botany. They went far towards disentangling a mass of confusing reports published during the previous ten years. And they helped considerably to support the notion of specific aetiology: the idea that particular infections are caused by particular microbes, which do not vary between one case and another and which can be isolated for study in the laboratory.

Koch and his postulates

There is another reason to remember Ferdinand Cohn. He encouraged the second outstanding experimentalist who, along with Louis Pasteur, established specific aetiology as the principle axis of modern medical science. Robert Koch was born in Hanover in 1843 and, after qualifying in medicine, served with the army throughout the Franco-Prussian war. In 1872 he was appointed district medical officer in Wollstein, a small town in Polish Prussia. There he began to pursue bacteriological research in a simple laboratory in his small house. One condition he tackled was anthrax. By the spring of 1876 he felt that he had solved the major problems of its aetiology, but needed advice about what to do next. So he approached Cohn. 'Esteemed Professor,' he wrote, 'I would be most grateful if you, as a leading authority on bacteria, would give me your criticism of my work before I submit it for publication.' Although Cohn received many communications from dilettantes, and felt pessimistic about such a letter from an unknown doctor in an obscure town, he nevertheless agreed to Koch's request to visit him in Breslau to demonstrate his experiments.

'Within the very first hour I recognised that he was an unsurpassed master of scientific research,' wrote Cohn of his feelings during that initial meeting. Cohn invited other observers for the subsequent days of demonstration and afterwards sent Koch home in a highly elated state. Koch's written report of his work—remembered today as a classic—was complete three weeks later, and Cohn published it in the new journal he was editing. He continued to help Koch and, indeed, established him on the scientific career for which he is now renowned.

What marked out Koch's labours as of abnormal significance was the punctiliousness he applied in proving his case. In 1849 Franz Pollender had seen microscopic bacilli in cattle that had died of anthrax, and in 1868 Casimir Davaine showed that the organisms were infectious. As little as one millionth of a drop of infected blood, he found, was enough to transmit the disease. And the number of organisms in blood samples apparently varied according to the severity of the attack.

Robert Koch did two things. First he discovered that anthrax bacilli produced spores, which were exceedingly resistant to heat and other adverse conditions. Provided that the temperature and amount of oxygen were right, spores always formed in the blood and tissues of animals that had died of the disease. This explained the persistence of anthrax and its reappearance in infected countryside: the spores could survive in the soil, causing infection many years later.

The other, crucial move by Robert Koch was to insist on a list of stringent requirements, each of which must be met before an organism could be incriminated positively as the agent of a particular disease. Now known as 'Koch's postulates', this was the set of conditions he applied to his own research on anthrax and, later, tuberculosis. Koch's starting-point was earlier work by Jakob Henle, under whom he had studied at Göttingen. In 1840, Henle had published a treatise entitled *Pathologische Untersuchungen*, which contained the first theoretical statement of the principles of specific aetiology. Henle divided epidemic diseases into three types: those transmitted by miasma (noxious effluvia in the atmosphere), those conveyed by contagion, and those whose primary origin was miasmatic but was followed by the development in the body of living parasites able to multiply and infect others. Henle noted the similarity between putrefaction and disease. Linking the work of Bassi and Caignard-Latour, he reasoned that smallpox pus must contain a living organism, and that the existence of different 'miasmatic-contagious' diseases implied the existence of different species of contagion.

Jakob Henle then explained what knowledge and techniques would be needed to prove that a specific infectious microorganism caused a particular disease. The suspect agent would have to be isolated in a pure state and recreate the disease again in an experimental animal. But the technical means of doing this were not yet available. And spontaneous generation, though doubted by Henle himself, was still an open question. That being so, his work is remarkable in setting out, largely from theory, the notion of specific aetiology and the requirements for its vindication.

The rules Koch formulated, each of which must be satisfied before a microorganism could be named conclusively as the agent of an infection, are that:

(a) A specific organism must invariably be associated with all cases of the disease.

(b) The organism must be isolated in pure culture and then subcultured over repeated generations.

(c) When inoculated into a healthy susceptible animal, the organism must again cause the disease.

(d) The organism must again be isolated in pure culture from the lesions of the disease.

The first condition, alone, is not enough. Such an association gave the earliest clues that the anthrax bacillus caused anthrax, as it provided the first pointers for Louis Pasteur in his studies on diseases of wine and beer. But as the sole indication of cause and effect it can be misleading. Many errors have resulted when microbiologists have adhered to this rule alone. Most spectacular was the wrongful implication of a bacterium, *Haemophilus influenzae*, as the agent of influenza more than thirty years before the real culprit (a much simpler form of life called a virus) was identified. To abide strictly by the other three rules, one requires sophisticated laboratory procedures for isolating suspect organisms in pure culture—cultures containing a single type of microbe rather than the heterogeneous community in which microorganisms usually occur.

Robert Koch could not satisfy his postulates fully in his anthrax work because these techniques were not yet to hand. But they were on the way. In 1872 Oscar Brefeld isolated and cultivated individual fungal spores, as a means of initiating pure cultures. Then in 1878 Lister showed that by diluting successively a suspension of bacteria he reached a dilution of which individual drops contained single organisms. Koch took these ideas much further and introduced laboratory skills that revolutionised the young subject of bacteriology. After his anthrax research was published he was appointed to the Imperial Health Office in Berlin, where he began work with Georg Gaffky and Friedrich Loeffler. Together they developed methods of growing colonies of bacteria first on the surface of potatoes and then on gelatine and agar. These techniques greatly facilitated the positive identification of pathogenic microbes, and Koch used them extensively in his most famous work, on tuberculosis, the definitive account of which was published in 1884. In that meticulous paper—dealing with a disease which killed one in every seven people at that time—Koch established the truth of specific aetiology beyond all reasonable doubt.

The immediate hope was that this would lead to appropriate cures for the infections whose causes were now being revealed.

But the first rewards were not with a drug but a vaccine, and with a disease we now know to be extraordinary in responding to immunisation *after* being contracted. This early success came to a lucky Pasteur—lucky in this instance because he was able to secure practical results without having met Robert Koch's stringent requirements. The malady was rabies. In 1881 Louis Pasteur and his colleagues reported changes in the central nervous system which they had seen in animals with the disease. Pasteur became convinced that a microbe was responsible. And because rabies seemed to have an unusually long incubation period he hoped to be able to protect people against the terrible symptoms by using attenuated organisms, as he had done with anthrax and fowl cholera.

But all attempts to cultivate an infective agent failed. So Pasteur decided instead to use spinal cord tissue from a rabid dog. He assumed this must contain the microbe. Injecting tissue that had been aged for progressively shorter times, he managed to immunise a dog for the first time in 1884—giving initially the well aged material, followed by successively less attenuated preparations, before challenging the dog with virulent rabies. Then on 6 July 1885 he concluded the earliest effective treatment of human rabies, in a little Alsatian boy, Joseph Meister. That was eighteen years before cell damage caused by rabies virus was observed directly and thirty years before animal viruses were cultivated. Pasteur's genius is illustrated again by this work, in which he retained faith in the concept of specific aetiology though rejecting for the moment the need to satisfy the practical tests laid down by Robert Koch. 'For him', René Dubos has said, 'doctrines and techniques were tools, to be used only as long as they lent themselves to the formulation and performance of meaningful experiments.'

The magic serum

Between 1879 and 1900, the causative agents of at least

twenty-two infections were discovered. Towards the end of the century, it seemed that microorganisms might be isolated from almost all diseases. Thus was born the high promise of specific therapy. As, one by one, microbes were indicted as pathogens, the prospect of fabricating corresponding chemical weapons to deal with them became compelling. The man who more than any other symbolises this hope and brought it to consummation was Paul Ehrlich. Born in Silesia in 1854—the year Pasteur went to Lille— Ehrlich qualified as a doctor at Leipzig and in 1887 became Reader in Medicine at the University of Berlin. Three years later Robert Koch provided him with a laboratory in the Institute for Infectious Diseases, to which he had moved in 1885. There and in other establishments in Steglitz and Frankfurt-am-Main he initiated the research which gave man power to combat infectious diseases with chemical missiles.

Ehrlich was an energetic man, an extrovert, who worked hard but enjoyed the good life too. He smoked twenty-five cigars a day and drank beer avidly. He also wrote more than 150 scientific papers, all containing evidence of his genius as well as his ingenuity in developing technical methods of experimentation. His first success was in bringing rigour and precision into the use of a newly devised weapon against diphtheria. Friedrich Loeffler had suspected that toxins (poisons), secreted by the bacilli, were responsible for the characteristic features of diphtheria. But he had not been able to prove his point. Then Émile Roux and Alexandre Yersin, at the newly created Institut Pasteur in Paris, showed that liquid in which the bacteria had been grown, filtered to remove all organisms, produced the typical lesions of diphtheria—and death—when injected into guinea-pigs. The toxin theory was vindicated. Shortly afterwards reports came from Robert Koch's laboratory that animals given repeated non-lethal doses of diphtheria toxin developed something in their serum that was capable of neutralising the poison. The same happened with tetanus. And the relationship was specific. The diphtheria 'antitoxin' reacted only with diphtheria toxin, not with tetanus toxin.

Tetanus antitoxin had no effect on the diphtheria poison.

So why not use antitoxin to treat the disease? One of Koch's assistants, Emil von Behring, set out to do so, having prepared antiserum by injecting diphtheria toxin into sheep and goats. The first time antiserum was used in treatment was on Christmas night 1891, when it was given to a child in a Berlin clinic.

The initial results with diphtheria antitoxin were dramatic. But success was short-lived. Soon it became obvious that this new weapon had to be deployed with care and calculation. Above all, the correct dose must be used, and several research workers tried to evolve the necessary methods of standardising antitoxins. They failed. This was where Paul Ehrlich's contribution was of paramount importance. A paper he published in 1897, one of the classic works in the science of immunology, contains the guidelines for standardising bacterial toxins and antitoxins as they are still followed to this day. It was based on laborious research, guided by Ehrlich's insistence on mathematical exactitude in matching toxin with antitoxin. As his measure for toxin, Ehrlich adopted the 'minimal lethal dose' — the smallest amount that would kill a guinea-pig weighing 250 grammes within four days. His unit of immunity was the quantity of antiserum that neutralised 100 times the minimum lethal dose of toxin in a 250-gramme guinea-pig. If these doses of toxin and antitoxin were injected simultaneously, the animal survived.

This groundwork was essential before diphtheria antitoxin* could be made available routinely and safely. When it did go into general use, about 1895, the consequences were dazzling. Within ten years the mortality rate for all types of diphtheria declined to less than half what it was beforehand. In London's fever hospitals the rate for laryngeal diphtheria in 1894 was 62 per cent; by 1910 it had fallen to under 12 per cent.

Paul Ehrlich's twin achievement in immunology was to show

---

*Not to be confused with toxoid, introduced forty years later for *immunisation* against diphtheria.

that antitoxin manufacture by animals is a widespread phenomenon. In 1891 he injected the vegetable poisons ricin and abrin into rabbits and found that antitoxins appeared in the bloodstream which were specific to the poisons. There was a 'latent period' before the antidotes developed, but the rabbits could then tolerate what otherwise would have been a fatal dose of the corresponding toxin. Ehrlich tried to explain in chemical terms what was happening. He envisaged that cells in the body carried 'receptors', to which toxin molecules could attach, poisoning the cells. Combined receptor and toxin was then shed into the bloodstream. In some circumstances, however, when an animal was immunised with a vaccine or tiny doses of a toxin, the cells fabricated excess receptors. These passed into the blood. There they circulated and were able to neutralise invading microbes and toxins before these could latch on to the cells and harm them. This was the earliest notion of 'antibodies', formed against 'antigens' in the invaders. Though Ehrlich's interpretation has been modified in the light of greater knowledge, it was the one which guided the development of modern immunology.

Towards chemotherapy

As the new science got under way, its exponents soon realised that not all infections behaved, or could be dealt with, like diphtheria. Serum from animals immunised against certain pathogens did not carry an antitoxin capable of neutralising a bacterial toxin. It disarmed the offending agents in a different manner. With cholera, for example, something in the immune serum attacked the cholera bacilli directly, breaking them down. And sera of this type proved to be disappointing or totally ineffective in treating conditions in the way tetanus and diphtheria antitoxins were used against tetanus and diphtheria. For many of man's other scourges — tuberculosis, cholera, typhoid fever — the main hope continued to rest in vaccines. Thus Robert Koch in 1891 introduced 'tuberculin', an extract prepared from dead tubercle bacilli, which he believed might cure the disease. But it was not a success and only in 1906 did two Frenchmen, Albert Calmette and Camille Guérin, perfect an attenuated vaccine (containing weakened bacteria) to use against tuberculosis. It was named BCG.

So the microbe hunters saw a crying need for weapons to deploy directly to vanquish the newly incriminated agents of disease. The answer came from a fusion between two of Paul Ehrlich's lines of research. While still a student, he had employed aniline dyes to render tiny objects visible under the microscope. One way he used them was to discover the various types of white blood cells. In 1881 he introduced methylene blue stain, which Robert Koch exploited in discovering the tubercle bacillus. Ehrlich then devised something even better, a stain that was highly specific to the tubercle bacillus. He also evolved a staining method for differentiating typhoid fever bacteria from similar-looking organisms. But Ehrlich began to realise that these dyes could be more than laboratory tools; they might also provide a specific means of attacking dangerous microbes in the body. At the same time, his work on antitoxins persuaded him that the body could harbour materials that were lethal to particular microorganisms yet harmless in every other way. Ehrlich compared these antibodies to 'magic bullets' which homed in on their target of their own accord and injured nothing else. So he set out on a quest to find chemicals which would destroy specific germs in the body but be otherwise innocuous.

Ehrlich's earliest attempt at what became known as 'chemotherapy' was simply by using methylene blue. In 1891 he administered it to a patient with malaria, and he considered the result beneficial—though this appears to have been uncertain. The first certain triumph came in 1907, when, after screening numerous benzo-purpurin dyes, he managed to cure the disease *mal de Caderas* in mice with trypan red. In the interim, his attention had been diverted from dyes to organic compounds containing arsenic. Researchers at the London School of Tropical Medicine had found that one such substance, atoxyl, was effective in combating trypanosome infections in animals. Ehrlich repeated this work, but discovered that if the dose was too low the parasites quickly became resistant to the drug. So he and his team of chemists started to synthesise innumerable variations on the atoxyl molecule, in the hope that one would prove much more potent and not meet the problem of resistance.

Success against syphilis

In 1905 Prussian, Fritz Schaudinn, identified the cause of syphilis, a thread-like organism now known as *Treponema pallidum*. Because of its similarity to the trypanosomes — and because of the toll of human suffering exacted by this parasite — Ehrlich began testing his synthetic substances against it too.

By 1907, Ehrlich's team had made and screened over 600 arsenic compounds. These varied enormously in their activity. One, No. 418, was particularly potent against the trypanosome infections. But none showed significant promise as drugs for dealing with syphilis. Then, in 1909, a Japanese bacteriologist, Sahachiro Hata, joined Ehrlich's group. He had specialised in investigating syphilis and had contrived to transmit it to rabbits, so Ehrlich asked him to test the entire series of arsenic compounds again to assess their action against *Treponema* in the rabbit. Hata found that one of them, No. 606, was both active and specific to the syphilis germ. During the previous trials one of Ehrlich's assistants had made an error in recording it as negative. The new drug, given the name Salvarsan, was first used to treat human syphilis in 1911. Disadvantages later came to light — principally its low solubility — and in due course Ehrlich devised the improved Neosalvarsan (compound No. 914).

These two magic bullets revolutionised the management of syphilis and heralded the arrival of chemotherapy — the specific chemical treatment of disease. Ehrlich was nominated for a Nobel Prize for this work in both 1912 and 1913. The nominations were not successful. The reason: he had already been awarded a Nobel Prize in 1908 for his achievements in immunology. Even then, the basis of his nomination had been disputed between those urging his various claims to fame; no scientist is expected to make so many major contributions to knowledge. Between 1901 and 1908, Ehrlich's name was put forward for a Nobel Prize seventy times, by thirteen different countries.

With only a handful of exceptions, such as quinine for malaria, all medical treatment for infectious disease up to the end of the nineteenth century was symptomatic — it ameliorated symptoms rather than attacked root causes. So the new prospect of chemotherapy was exciting and revolutionary. Louis Pasteur died in 1895 and shortly afterwards it seemed likely that, in his words, 'all parasitic maladies might be made to disappear from the face of the earth'.

The golden age

The era of chemotherapy — of antibiotics and synthetic anti-microbial drugs — did not arrive at once. But new magic bullets did come along, more and more of them, as the century progressed. In 1920 — five years after Ehrlich's death — chemists at the pharmaceutical firm of Bayer synthesised a drug, Bayer 205, which proved invaluable in combating human sleeping sickness. Synthetic improvements on quinine were introduced. Then came the 'sulpha drugs'. They began with a discovery in 1932 by Gerhard Domagk, working for I.G. Farbenindustrie. He found that the dye prontosil red controlled infections with streptococci (the agents of scarlet fever) in mice. The activity really stemmed from sulphanilamide, the substance to which the body converted prontosil red. Many other sulpha drugs were then fabricated — the best known being M & B 693. They produced near-miraculous cures for bacterial pneumonia, meningitis, puerperal fever, gonorrhoea, erysipelas, and bowel and urinary tract infections. Finally, the golden age of antibiotics arrived with Alexander Fleming's observations leading to the discovery of penicillin, made into a practical tool by Howard Florey and Ernst Chain in Oxford; and streptomycin, the 'wonder drug' for the treatment of tuberculosis, which was isolated by Selman Waksman in 1944. Chloramphenicol (a decisive weapon against typhoid fever), the tetracyclines, and many similar magic bullets have since come into use. Outstanding have been the 'new' penicillins, semi-synthetic drugs made by modifying the penicillin molecule chemically. They were introduced in the late 1950s by the Beecham group in the United Kingdom. Both the penicillins and the tetracyclines have come into widespread use against a wide range of infections, particularly respiratory and intestinal troubles.

Even greater precision

Meanwhile, specific aetiology was being pushed to new frontiers of discrimination. Gradually it became clear that infections like tuberculosis and diphtheria were not caused by single types of bacteria. Often there is a variety of different strains, each with its own distinctive behaviour. Typhoid fever is a classic example. In 1934, at the Lister Institute in London, Arthur Felix and Margaret Pitt were cross-testing typhoid bacilli with antibodies prepared against other strains. They found that the most virulent bacteria were distinct from the others, because they carried a characteristic antigen, now known as the Vi or virulence antigen. This can be used as a marker to identify particularly virulent forms of typhoid bacilli. The same technique is employed in hospital laboratories to study many other different categories of microorganisms. Some groups of bacteria contain hundreds of strains, each having individual characteristics.

In very recent years, specific aetiology has been taken further in another respect. Scientists now wish to know why particular organisms infect only particular species of animals or particular tissues. Why does the distemper virus attack dogs but not man? Why does influenza virus grow prolifically in the human respiratory tract but not in the tongue or liver? Research initiated in Britain at the Microbiological Research Establishment, Porton Down, has shed some light on these puzzles. The earliest breakthrough came in the 1960s during investigations into brucellosis by Dr Harry Smith and his colleagues. In many animals, including man, brucellosis is a relatively mild disease, and the bacteria responsible (brucellae) have no special affinity for one tissue or another. But in pregnant cows, sheep, goats, and sows, brucellae multiply massively in the foetal membranes and fluids. The result is abortion, a serious cause of economic loss in animal husbandry. The explanation which emerged from Harry Smith's work is that susceptible uterine tissue in vulnerable species contains erythritol, a 'sugar alcohol' that stimulates the invading brucellae to proliferate. In cattle, for example, the foetal placentae, membranes and fluids are a rich source of erythritol, whereas other tissues in the foetus and those of the mother contain little or none. This is why the bacteria produce their characteristic damage. And the absence of erythritol in the human placenta is the reason why brucellae do not cause abortion in man. Such a simple, precise demonstration of cause and effect would have delighted Robert Koch and the other nineteenth-century prophets of specific aetiology.

Vitamins and vitamin deficiency

As we have seen, specific aetiology was well attuned with the deterministic mood of science in the last century. After its early dividends in explaining infections, hopes grew that a diligent search would reveal the particular causes of all diseases. There was little progress at first, but then the concept was vindicated elegantly in two other, unrelated, fields. The first centred on the discovery of vitamins.

Christiaan Eijkman was the man who, between 1893 and 1897, made the crucial breakthrough that led to our present understanding of vitamins and the disorders caused by their deficiency. The son of a schoolmaster, Eijkman was born at Nijerk in Holland. He trained as a medical officer for the Army of the Dutch East Indies, and graduated in medicine from Amsterdam in 1883. A few years later the Dutch government sent a Commission to study beri-beri in Batavia (now Djakarta), following many severe outbreaks of the disease in colonies in Java and Sumatra. The Commission returned to Europe in 1887. But its laboratory, based at a military hospital, was kept in being and Eijkman became the director. By chance, during his continued experiments there, chickens reared in the laboratory developed a condition, characterised by paralysis, which resembled very closely beri-beri in man. As with the human disease, there was no evidence that an infectious microbe was the culprit. But Eijkman noticed that his assistant had been feeding the birds on cooked rice from the military hospital. When a new cook arrived — one who refused to allow the hospital's rice to be sent to the laboratory — the disease abated.

Christiaan Eijkman spotted the relevance of this and went on to show that he could precipitate the paralytic malady by feeding chickens on a diet consisting exclusively of polished rice, in place of unmilled rice. Moreover, the bran removed by polishing would cure the disease, even if given together with polished rice. A few years later, the active component was found to be a vitamin, the absence of which caused beri-beri. Now known as thiamin, this was the first of the B-group vitamins to be isolated. Experiments in the first decade of this century by Frederick Gowland Hopkins in Britain led to the discovery of other vitamins. He and Eijkman shared the Nobel Prize for Medicine and Physiology in 1929.

Among the diseases we now know to be attributable to shortage of a particular vitamin are: rickets, tetany, night blindness, scurvy, polyneuritis, pellagra, dermatitis and megaloblastic anaemia. Most of these conditions can be ameliorated simply by administering the corresponding vitamin. Such diseases, known as avitaminoses, thus represent chemical confirmation of specific aetiology.

Disease in the genes

A second group of conditions which afforded further authentication of the theory were hereditary defects. At the turn of the century, Archibald Garrod noted that four diseases were all present at birth and thereafter throughout life, occurred characteristically in families, and were more frequent in the offspring of consanguinous marriages. Albinism caused by defective pigmentation of the skin, hair and eyes, was one and the others were conditions in which bizarre chemicals appeared in the victims' urine. Garrod surmised correctly that they resulted from discrete faults in the genes controlling body chemistry. Today we recognise several of these 'inborn errors of metabolism'. In several of them, illness follows the accumulation of a substance in the body because of congenital absence of the enzyme that would normally have converted it into something else. One such disease is phenylketonuria. Untreated, it results in mental deficiency, abnormally light skin and hair pigmentation, and occasionally epilepsy. The underlying explanation is that those who inherit the defective gene lack an enzyme required to process phenylalanine — one of the constituent amino acids of protein. And the devastating syndrome can be avoided simply by ensuring that there is a very low concentration of this amino acid in the diet from the earliest possible age.

Cause-and-effect at this level reflects almost Calvinistic determinism. As J. B. S. Haldane has remarked, to say that 'John Smith is a complete fool because he cannot oxidise phenylalanine, discloses a relation between mind and matter as surprising as transubstantiation, and a good deal better established'. What it also does is to confirm again the fruitfulness of specific aetiology in explaining the basis of disease.

Hormones—further proof

Hot on the heels of Archibald Garrod, the Japanese biochemist Jokichi Takimine made a discovery which, in due course, strengthened the theory further still. He isolated adrenalin—the first hormone to be purified. That was in 1901, and twenty years later, in December 1921, another hormone, insulin, held the centre of the stage when Dr Frederick Banting and Dr Charles Best reported their historic work on its relationship to diabetes.

Banting was born in Alliston, Ontario, the son of a farmer. After qualifying in medicine at the University of Toronto in 1916 he served in the First World War and received the Military Cross for gallantry. When peace came he worked for a short time as a surgeon in London, Ontario. During those years he read an article about the apparent but still unclear relation of diabetes to the Islets of Langerhans. These are tiny accumulations of cells in the pancreas. Unlike the rest of the gland (which produces digestive juices) they were thought to secrete directly into the bloodstream a hormone concerned with regulating blood sugar. Banting reasoned that by tying up the ducts through which digestive juices leave the pancreas the entire gland except the islets would be destroyed. If the islets secreted a hormone, it could then be isolated.

In 1921, Banting asked the permission of Professor J. J. R. McLeod, head of the physiology department at the University of Toronto, to use his laboratory for the investigation. McLeod agreed and Banting began work. He was joined by Charles Best, a young American who had graduated recently in the department. McLeod was away from the laboratory during most of the months following, when Banting and Best made the crucial breakthrough. By the autumn of 1921 they had isolated insulin and established its specific role in preventing diabetes in dogs. In view of the importance of their discovery, Banting and Best were anxious not to have to wait for a report to appear in a learned journal. They hoped instead to describe their results at a meeting of the American Physiological

Society in December. As the Society had a rule that at least one member of a team presenting a paper must be a member, McLeod included his name on the communication — the other two not being members. When the paper was printed the following year, the three names appeared again.

At about the same time, Banting and Best had taken their work further. With the help of a young chemist, J. B. Collip, they had isolated enough insulin, of sufficient purity, to try on a human patient with diabetes. Just eighteen months after starting their investigation, they injected insulin into a diabetic — and it worked. The next year, Banting and McLeod received a Nobel Prize 'for their discovery of insulin'. Best's name was not mentioned. Banting was furious, and he shared his prize money with Best. Afterwards McLeod gave half of his money to Collip.

Sickle cell anaemia—one error in 300

Specific aetiology in its most precise form is exemplified by the work of Vernon Ingram at Cambridge, England, in the late 1950s on sickle cell anaemia. This is a hereditary condition, common among Negroes, in which the red blood cells cannot transport oxygen normally. Instead they become distorted into sickle-shapes. Most victims die in childhood, and those who survive suffer a chronic illness accompanied by painful crises when the blood supply is cut off from various organs in the body. There is no effective treatment. The reason why the disease has persisted in some populations is that the mutant gene responsible also confers resistance against malaria. That advantage explains why the mutation has not been eliminated through evolution.

The mutation is in the gene controlling the synthesis of haemoglobin, the protein in red blood cells which carries oxygen. Somehow the abnormal haemoglobin produced by the faulty gene cannot perform properly. Vernon Ingram set out to discover why. Which part of the molecule was defective?

The task seemed gargantuan, because haemoglobin is a complex molecule consisting of some 8,000 atoms. (Working out the complete structure had taken research workers at Cambridge nearly ten years.) However, the molecule is made up of two identical halves, each consisting of about 300 different amino acid units. So Dr Ingram and his colleagues had to break down haemoglobin into its constituent parts and compare sequences of amino acids in each region of the normal molecule with those in the sickle-cell version. They eventually found that just one amino acid differed in the two structures.

As Ingram wrote:

According to our evidence, the sole chemical difference is that in the abnormal molecule a valine is substituted for glutamic acid at one point. A change of one amino acid in nearly 300 is certainly a very small change indeed, and yet this slight alteration can be fatal to the unfortunate possessor of the errent haemoglobin. Equally remarkable is the fact that the sickle cell gene operates so delicately on the synthesis of a protein, changing just one amino acid and leaving the rest of the molecule's structure unaltered.

Such particularity is an uncanny vindication of the theory of specific aetiology.

The success of this approach to disease was symbolised by the appearance, late in 1976, of the first issue of a new journal, *Molecular Aspects of Medicine*, published by Pergamon. In their introduction the editors, Dr John Gergely of the Boston Biomedical Research Institute and Professor Harold Baum of Chelsea College, London, highlight the sickle cell research and also the discovery of isoenzymes — differing forms of the same enzyme, whose study has helped in pinpointing the site of pathological processes. An aim of the new journal is to 'generate new developments in the field of underlying biochemical and biological phenomena, which in turn will lead to a better understanding, and eventual solution, of clinical problems'.

Surgery on the psyche

With the exception of hereditary afflictions like phenylketonuria, mental illness has not presented such a fertile field as physical disease for specific aetiology. But as we shall see in more detail in Chapter 5, attempts have been made to explain and certainly to deal with mental illness in this way. The most dramatic of these has been psychosurgery: the destruction or removal of brain tissue with the intention of correcting abnormal behaviour. Its origins take us back to a Portuguese neurologist, Antonio Egas Moniz.

Moniz was born in Avanca. He gained his medical degree in 1899 at the University of Coimbra, where he became professor of neurology three years later and where he had previously taught mathematics. There he developed a keen interest in improving radiological methods for detecting brain tumours. Appointed to the chair of neurology at Lisbon in 1911, Moniz began to experiment with dyes, opaque to X-rays, which he injected into cadavers before taking X-ray pictures. The resulting plates revealed the position of the principal cerebral arteries. Next he moved on to living subjects — and to patients. By 1907 Moniz was able to determine the location and size of a pituitary tumour by examining the way in which arteries, injected with the dyes, were displaced. Some of the dyes later turned out to be toxic, but safe replacements were found and this technique has since become routine.

In 1935-6 Antonio Egas Moniz entered the field which brought him even greater fame. Moniz was one of the earliest and most determined supporters of the concept of organic, physical causes of — and thus treatments for — mental illness. That is how he came to learn of the flourishing school of neurophysiology at Yale University led by John Fulton, who was trying to learn where various mental functions were located in the brain of anthropoid apes. Attending the international neurological conference in London in 1935, Moniz heard that while John Fulton and his colleagues had induced artificial neuroses in normal, healthy apes, they found they could not do so in apes from which they had removed the frontal lobes of the brain. Chimpanzees with their frontal lobes isolated by the operation now known as leucotomy became markedly more friendly and docile. They no longer developed the violent tantrums which they formerly exhibited when making mistakes in solving psychological problems.

Another, totally fortuitous, event that contributed to the emerging understanding of brain function occurred in 1848 when an iron rod, over an inch thick, was accidentally driven through the head of Phineas Gage, a road construction worker in San Francisco. Gage was merely stunned, and within half an hour managed to walk—with the bar sticking through his left cheek and out the top of his head—to a surgeon for help. Despite an infection of the sort then so common after surgery, Gage recovered well. He lived for another twelve years and died from causes unrelated to his head injury.

What was most intriguing, however, was the subtle change in Phineas Gage's personality after the incident. He became 'restless, obstinate, profane, lax about work and inconsiderate of the feeling of others', having previously been both mild and considerate. His intellect deteriorated slightly, but his memory and ability to work seemed unimpaired. After Gage's death, an autopsy showed that the left frontal lobe of his brain was largely destroyed. There was also some injury to the right frontal lobe. This evidence, and later observations on patients with other sorts of brain damage, including tumours, showed that personality changes were the most common sequel to frontal lobe injury—which at the time had no effect on vital bodily processes.

Moniz reasoned that in forms of mental illness characterised by extreme emotional tension some of the nerve paths arising in the frontal lobes were excessively active, so that messages were transmitted repeatedly, thereby gaining undue precedence. Such individuals might be helped by having these nerve paths severed. Moniz carried out his first tests on human patients in a Lisbon mental institution, isolating the frontal lobes by injecting alcohol into the connecting white matter of the brain. The results were considered highly successful. Of the first twenty patients, seven were declared cured and eight improved. None of them died.

Antonio Egas Moniz was not the first person to operate on the human brain, but formerly this had been done only in cases of organic disease. Moniz was the first to tamper with the brain in an attempt to correct specific psychological aberration. His work is a surgical parallel of 'selective toxicity—the idea that one can destroy parasites in the body by using magic bullets that leave the patient's tissues unharmed (or broadcast insecticides to kill insects without hurting man, or destroy weeds with weedkillers without damaging crops). Underlying the strategy of selective toxicity is the theory of specific aetiology. This has been one of the most powerful and productive tools in the history of medicine. Yet, as we shall see, it also has its disappointments, drawbacks, and dangers.

4
The failure of a theory

Around 1900, when he was 74, a Bavarian doctor, Max von Pettenkofer, knowingly consumed a culture containing millions of cholera bacilli, isolated from a fatal case of the disease. At about the same time the Russian pathologist Elie Metchnikoff conducted the same bizarre experiment. So did several of their colleagues. Some of the intrepid experimenters experienced mild diarrhoea. All had enormous numbers of cholera bacilli in their faeces. But none developed anything like cholera.

Von Pettenkofer, like Koch, Pasteur, and Ehrlich, was one of the pioneers in the study of infection. But he refused to be converted to the germ theory of disease; he believed instead in 'poisonous miasmata'. So when Robert Koch returned from a trip to India, where he had discovered the cholera germ, his Bavarian critic was happy to put his own disbelief to the test. Today, von Pettenkofer is remembered as a founder of modern hygiene. Metchnikoff is celebrated as the discoverer of phagocytes, the white blood cells which can engulf and destroy invading germs. His life's work centred upon the healing power of the body in its battles against infection. Metchnikoff's researches were taken further in Britain by Almroth Wright, who was caricatured as Sir Colenso Rigeon in Bernard Shaw's play *The Doctor's Dilemma*. Wright headed the department of St Mary's Hospital, London, where Alexander Fleming observed the action of penicillin, and his influence may well have contributed to Fleming's failure to capitalise on his good fortune. Metchnikoff and Wright both taught that the correct way to deal with infectious disease was not by administering chemicals but by strengthening and where necessary exploiting the body's own defences.

One thing was abundantly clear, however, from the demonstrations of von Pettenkofer and Metchnikoff. Specific aetiology had suffered a severe blow. Until that point, the microbe hunters had been confidently isolating microorganisms from one infection after another, injecting them into animals, and reproducing corresponding diseases. Using Koch's postulates, they were then able to establish cause and effect. The ease and predictability with which they did so contrasted starkly with the failure of two great experimenters to give themselves cholera — and indeed with many subsequent attempts to produce infectious disease in man. So marked is the difference between the work of the laboratory and the real world that the triumphs of Pasteur and Koch seem virtually incompatible with nature.

The paradox is explained by the highly artificial conditions used in most of the early experiments. René Dubos explains:

> Pasteur and Koch did not deal with natural events, but with experimental artefacts. The experimenter does not reproduce nature in the laboratory. He could not if he tried, for the experiment imposes limiting conditions on nature; its aims are to force nature to give answers to questions devised by man. Every answer of nature is therefore more or less influenced by the kind of questions asked.

This does not mean that specific aetiology is untrue. It *does* suggest that the notion is simplistic, and that much more needs to be taken into account in delineating the essence of disease. Nutrition, environment, Hippocratic 'constitution', age, and many other factors determine the pattern of infectious maladies and individual susceptibility to them. According to the great British physician James Paget, 'fatigue has a larger share in the promotion and transmission of disease than any other single condition you can name', and today it also appears that the body's natural biological rhythms influence the course of illnesses. In contrast with such vague factors, spectacular claims of cause and effect provide a tempting certainty. That is why specific aetiology—despite the courageous self-experiments of von Pettenkofer and Metchnikoff—has exerted a disproportionate influence on the development of medical research and practice. But the theory in all its simple elegance is wrong. In this chapter we shall see why.

Infection is not disease

Before examining the failure of specific aetiology in accounting for coronary heart disease, cancer, and mental illness, which loom so large today, we shall scrutinise more closely its utility in accounting for infectious disease—the sector of medicine in which it arose and received its first accolades. The earliest doubts came when the categorical division of microbes into pathogens and non-pathogens began to look suspect. As bacteriologists refined their methods of examining and testing microorganisms, it became clear that immense numbers of genuinely pathogenic varieties could be recovered from individuals who were in excellent health. During epidemics of meningitis, many people harboured the causative agents without suffering detectable illness. Often, a greater proportion of healthy folk could be found carrying the germs than those who developed meningitis. This was not simply because they had developed antibodies during an earlier bout of meningitis. Precisely the same virulent bacteria, infecting non-immune individuals, will produce disease in some and not in others. And on balance the relationship between man and microbe favours peaceful coexistence rather than open warfare.

Modern techniques are a good deal more discriminating than they were in Pasteur's day, and they have allowed bacteriologists to demonstrate such differences experimentally. Professor G. T. Stewart, for example, at the University of North Carolina, has shown that distinct strains of laboratory animals vary widely in their response to injection with a standard quantity of tubercle bacilli. In man, one way of studying this phenomenon is to compare the medical records of large numbers of twins — identical twins, who were derived from one egg cell and thus share exactly the same genes; and non-identical twins, who originated by the fertilisation of two different egg cells. Such studies have revealed surprising contrasts. For example, an identical twin in the United States has a three out of four chance of developing tuberculosis if the other twin has the clinical disease, whereas a non-identical twin has a chance of only one in three. Ethnic origin plays a role too. Tuberculosis, rheumatic fever and pneumonia are strikingly more prevalent and severe in American Negroes than Whites — even when allowance is made for socioeconomic differences.

Behaviour, including its apparently trivial aspects, also has a real effect on individual susceptibility to disease. Mouth breathers, nose pickers, and heavy smokers are more prone to respiratory infections than those who do not adopt, or who relinquish, these habits. Similarly, scratching, excessive washing and use of deodorants and other toiletries encourage skin infection by obliterating protective bacteria and thus lowering the skin's natural resistance. Venereal disease provides the clearest example of the effect of behaviour. A public health programme founded securely on specific aetiology, and designed to eradicate syphilis simply by exploiting its sensitivity to penicillin, would be doomed to failure. The real determinant here is human behaviour.

Most of those in the audience on 24 March 1882 at the meeting of the Physiological Society in Berlin when Robert Koch announced his discovery of the tubercle bacillus had undoubtedly been parasitised by this germ at some stage in their lives. Many probably still carried the virulent bacilli in their bodies. At that time, virtually all city dwellers in Europe were infected with *Mycobacterium tuberculosis*. Yet only a tiny proportion suffered in any way as a result. Koch himself had been invaded. He proved this in 1890, when he injected tuberculin into his arm and suffered a violent reaction—a sure sign that the tubercle bacillus had multiplied in his tissues earlier in his life. But Koch was fit and hearty, remaining so until he died after a stroke at the age of sixty-six. In a situation of this sort— universal infection, but infrequent disease—the real cause of tuberculosis is not the bacillus but the malnutrition, fatigue and other accompaniments of poverty which turn harmless parasitism into overt ill health.

Koch and Pasteur, however, wanted to prove that micro-organisms caused specific diseases. Their genius was in devising experiments which unequivocally supported that hypothesis. They stacked all the odds in their favour by finding, after trial and error, animals and methods of inoculation which produced the right result unfailingly. They thus minimised all of those environmental and bodily factors which might modify microbial malevolence. In their classic demonstrations, it was sufficient to arrange for an encounter between pathogen and susceptible rabbit or guinea-pig to make the outcome certain.

One of the most famous and apparently clear-cut incidents in the conquest of infectious disease happened in 1854 when Dr John Snow demanded that the handle be removed from the public water pump in Broad Street, London. A cholera epidemic was raging in the capital which had caused 500 deaths in ten days in one small area alone. After making house-to-house inquiries, Snow realised that all of the victims had collected their drinking water from the same Broad Street pump. So the handle was disconnected—and a few days later the epidemic abated. Yet many people, doctors included, remained unmoved. They were more impressed by the observation that cholera, like tuberculosis, was invariably associated with filthy living conditions.

We still do not understand in detail what turns infection with the cholera germ into a devastating disease. Nutrition is important, as is the moment of infection and the level of acidity in an individual's stomach at the time. To do their worst, the organisms must pass through the acid and into the lower intestine. Even after arriving there, however, they do not necessarily provoke disease — as von Pettenkofer and Metchnikoff showed with such panache. Koch's first postulate, it seems, is in need of modification. True, there is no tuberculosis without *Mycobacterium tuberculosis*, no syphilis or cholera without their corresponding microbes. But the reverse reasoning is invariably erroneous. Streptococci, poliomyelitis viruses, the pneumococci responsible for pneumonia, and other 'pathogens' may be carried for many months without doing any harm to their hosts.

So too with Koch's further postulates. The disease, if any, caused when an experimentalist injects a pathogen into an animal is determined as much by the recipient as by the microbe. The postulates are not erroneous, but seriously incomplete. In Professor Stewart's words:

> They fail to allow for biological variations and they make no allowance for the complex conditions influencing infection in natural settings; they are narrowly adapted to defining rigid conditions which happen to fit the behaviour of a few microorganisms studied on limited lines by Koch and others in a few susceptible hosts; but from this narrow basis, the postulates were stretched to form a theory with a general applicability to all infectious diseases.

The dramatic demonstrations of Pasteur and the meticulous laboratory experiments of Koch were basically artefacts, giving a highly distorted impression of how microbes behave in nature.

Publication of Charles Creighton's *History of Epidemics in Britain* in 1894 did something to counter the advances of the specific aetiologists, by stimulating renewed interest in the natural history of disease, in the Hippocratic tradition. Then the gradual recognition that perfectly fit individuals could and often did harbour large numbers of pathogens during epidemics without contracting disease was extended by the work of Percival Horton-Smith. In his Goulstonian Lectures of

1900, Horton-Smith described an apparently healthy person who excreted the typhoid bacillus in his urine. This was the first report of the 'carrier state'. Little attention was paid at first to Horton-Smith's and similar accounts (though the discovery later became important in measures to prevent the spread of typhoid fever). Despite increasing evidence that disease was not the inevitable result of a collision between parasite and host, the simpler view prevailed. It has dominated the evolution of medicine to this day.

Rich man, poor man

Nutrition is a major factor which specific aetiology ignores. In the real world, it is crucially important in determining the course of infectious disease. Measles, for example, is a virtually universal infection in all social classes. But the chances of serious illness—and of death—depend largely on the general health of a child. Nutrition and past illnesses influence the outcome greatly, making measles vastly more dangerous among the poor. We know too from experience in German concentration camps during the Second World War that, with emaciation, harmless infection can become severe skin disease or bronchopneumonia. (Most internees who returned to their normal environment after the war recovered rapidly from such afflictions without the help of specific therapy.) But the relation between nutrition and infection is complex. It can be tantalisingly difficult to unravel in a community where people are both poor (and thus underfed) and overcrowded (and thus greatly exposed to infections such as tuberculosis or, in a tropical country, schistosomiasis*). And there is two-way interaction. Malnutrition makes it easier for parasites to invade the body and establish themselves. It also retards convalescence. Conversely, infectious disease adversely affects nutrition. It does so both directly, impairing appetite and interfering with

*Formerly known as bilharzia (see p. 191).

the absorption of food, and indirectly by encouraging parents to give sick children a 'simpler', less nutritious diet and/or to administer purgatives. The result is a vicious circle, seen all too clearly in conditions of poverty and underdevelopment. The World Health Organisation claims that a combination of malnutrition and infection accounts for between half and three-quarters of all statistically recorded deaths of infants and young children.

The lack of nourishment is rarely specific. Avitaminoses such as beri-beri and rickets do occur, but much more commonly the condition is chronic and non-specific. In some countries two-thirds of the population are affected and, while an infectious microorganism is almost always the eventual cause of death, the real explanation of high mortality is the lack of proper food. A field study conducted in four Guatemalan villages by the WHO in 1956-7 showed that a third of the deaths in children from one to four years old were from malnutrition, usually with a precipitating infection. Almost another third of the children died of acute diarrhoeal disease — which is rarely fatal to a well fed child. Most of the remainder succumbed to respiratory disease, often as a complication of measles, chickenpox or whooping cough. Again, such fatalities are unusual among children who are well nourished. Doctors in developed countries rarely see this association of afflictions. Before vaccination, almost every infant in every country in the world contracted measles. But there were 300 times more deaths from the disease, per child, in the poorer nations than in the rich ones. According to a 1974 report by the WHO, 'we have given too much attention to the enemy and have to some extent overlooked our own defences . . . For the time being, an adequate diet is the most effective 'vaccine' against most of the diarrhoeal, respiratory and other common infections.'

These comments may not apply to all infections. Thomas Sydenham reported that smallpox plagued the well off rather than the destitute, and the same was probably true of the 'English sweats'—a mysterious fever which ravaged England during Tudor times and whose cause has still not been established with certainty. The adequately fed fared least well too in the 1918-19 pandemic of influenza. Edwin Chadwick, the English barrister and leading activist in promoting preventive medicine in the mid-nineteenth century, also discovered the greatest amount of disease and the highest death rate among well nourished captives in the country's gaols. But the prisoners with the worst health were poor agricultural workers shortly after going into prison — which may be explained by the change from a near-starvation diet to prison fare. Two American doctors, M. J. Murray and A. B. Murray, from the University of Minnesota, have put forward a hypothesis to explain this paradox. Perhaps starvation suppresses certain infections, while refeeding activates them. This could be part of an ecological balance between *Homo sapiens* and his environment. Man fails to thrive during famine, but the fecundity of his 'micropredators' declines in parallel. In times of plenty, the corresponding increase in the parasites acts as a check against excessive human multiplication. The Murrays' thesis is controversial, and one of its weaknesses is its apparent application to some serious human infections but not others. It does, however, square with a good deal of evidence — and certainly confirms that there is still much to learn about the association between nutrition and ill health.

Magic bullets—two-edged weapons

Nearly a century on, then, specific aetiology looks somewhat tattered — even in the sector of medicine that saw its first thrilling conquests. So what of those strategies of warfare against infectious disease which have been, and still are, largely based on this theory? The picture is not impressive. As recently as October 1976, participants at an international symposium held at Limburg, West Germany, concluded that within the next twenty years antibiotics may be looked upon as 'a useful but temporary and historic form of treatment'. Professor W. A. Altemeier, from the University of Cincinnati, argued that antibiotics had made wound infection more difficult, not easier, to manage. Resistant strains of bacteria were to blame, and life-threatening complications were becoming commoner. His and other speakers' contributions threw into sharp relief the contrast between what is now considered an old-fashioned means of combating infectious disease — by prevention, by hygiene, and by aseptic precautions to thwart infection during surgery — and the 'modern' approach which trusts heavily in the potency of magic bullets. That dependence now appears increasingly foolhardy amidst an inexorable, world-wide proliferation of drug resistant strains of bacteria.

The earliest indications that magic bullets might be two-edged weapons came when the first antibiotics were deployed in massive doses with careless abandon. The repercussions included vitamin deficiencies, vaginal thrush, and yeast infections of the intestine. These results followed the indiscriminate slaughter of pathogens and helpful organisms too — those which normally protect the body against invaders. The balanced relationship between man and his microbes had been shattered.

We have not learned from these mistakes. Doctors still prescribe antibiotics for trivial maladies as well as serious ones. Potent drugs which should be reserved to treat really serious infections are available freely across the counter in many countries. And farmers have been allowed to put some of the same substances in feedstuffs to make their pigs, calves and broiler fowls grow more quickly. The consequence of all this has been a menacing spread of bacteria which are invulnerable to antibiotics. Thus epidemics of untreatable disease, produced by bacteria insensitive to the drugs that could otherwise have been used in therapy, have become increasingly common.

Bacteria can become resistant to antibiotics and other magic bullets in two different ways. They may mutate. One organism in many millions develops the new skill — and gains a corresponding advantage over susceptible cells in the presence of the drug concerned. Frequent and indiscriminate use of the drugs — giving them in the wrong doses and for conditions where they are not really needed—encourages the emergence of a resistant population. The other sort of resistance is even more worrying. Discovered by Japanese bacteriologists in 1959, this is transferable resistance, resistance that can spread from one organism to another. It is often multiple (sensitive bacteria may acquire resistance to as many as seven or eight drugs at a time) and is particularly common among microorganisms that colonise the gut, including dysentery and typhoid fever bacilli. The ability can be transmitted freely between pathogens and non-pathogens in the intestine. Thus a 'pool' of resistance builds up in the gut flora which may at any time be passed on to virulent organisms.

Transferable resistance is a natural phenomenon. We have turned it into a serious problem. Family practitioners handing out antibiotics for mild infections which would clear up themselves without treatment, farmers deploying the drugs in vast quantities in livestock feeds, surgeons trusting in massive doses to cover their patients against infection during operations—all these have contributed to the current situation. As the Limburg conference implied, we are moving back rapidly to pre-antibiotic days. The antimicrobial armouries upon which we have come to rely have been disarmed. In many ways we are worse off than before, possession of the 'wonder drugs' having made us negligent of natural methods of healing. How many of those of us who should take a couple of days in bed to shake off a heavy cold or chest infection are encouraged not to do so by the belief that antibiotics are available if anything goes badly wrong? How many demand penicillin or similar from our doctor anyway, and thus interfere with the body's usually adequate capacity for self-restoration?

The consequences of the free deployment of antibiotics grow more disquieting year by year. The first deeply worrying reports came from E. S. Anderson, at the Enteric Reference Laboratory, Colindale, London, in the 1960s. He discovered a huge rise in drug resistance following the massive application of ampicillin and other drugs to prevent disease during the intensive rearing of calves—something which could and should be done by improving the conditions of husbandry. Outbreaks of human food-poisoning were linked with this growth in resistance; the bacteria responsible pass freely between animals and man. Similar evidence came from Holland. More recently, chloramphenicol-resistant typhoid bacilli have thrived dramatically in Mexico, India, Thailand and Vietnam. Chloramphenicol is virtually the only drug that is effective against typhoid fever (it should be reserved for this use only), and resistant strains infected some 100,000 patients in Mexico around 1974, killing 14,000 of them. Ampicillin-resistant *Haemophilus influenzae* has begun to cause untreatable meningitis among children in the USA, while food-poisoning salmonellae invulnerable to several drugs have been found in Portugal, Belgium, Canada and Israel. 'The time has come', Professor Anderson warned recently, 'when international co-operation at legislative and professional levels is needed to attempt to reverse the change in the ecology of the enterobacteria and other organisms that has resulted from the indiscriminate use of antibacterial drugs.'

Mistaken therapy

The positive value of antibiotics should not be minimised. While they are often given without good cause, they are of undeniable practical importance. Among intestinal infections, for example, not only typhoid fever but also *Salmonella* food poisoning may require antibiotic therapy especially in the very old, the very young, and the malnourished. What is wrong is that many doctors (and many patients too) know nothing like enough about such drugs to use these potent—and dangerous—weapons properly. One illustration of this comes from a televised 'National Antibiotic Therapy Test' held in the USA in 1975. An audience of 4,500 doctors joined in the project, which was designed to assess their competence in diagnosing and treating infectious disease. Both family practitioners and specialists took part. Simulated clinical problems were presented, followed by questions about how they should be handled.

The results were striking. Only two of the 4,500 participants achieved full marks. One entrant contrived to register a score that was below par for guessing. Competence was compared by calculating the percentage of doctors in the different categories with a mark of 80 per cent or more. On this basis, family practitioners recorded 15 per cent and surgeons 10 per cent. Paediatricians (24 per cent) and internal medicine specialists (38 per cent) did somewhat better, but the only respectable rating was that of infectious diseases specialists (83 per cent). And the questions were all on topics which any doctor prescribing antimicrobial drugs should know about, such as when to give chloramphenicol, and what other medicines sulpha drugs may interact with.

There was also serious ignorance of how to employ laboratory services. The correct way to prescribe antibiotics is for the doctor to take a throat swab or other specimen which he then sends to the pathology laboratory. There the infectious organism is identified and its antibiotic sensitivity assessed so that the practitioner knows which drug to administer. But many doctors do not bother with these facilities, or use them haphazardly. One investigation which showed this was reported by Dr R. J. Taylor and his colleagues in Aberdeen, Scotland, in 1975. They found that the number of vaginal swabs, faecal specimens, throat swabs and urine specimens submitted by 104 practitioners to the local bacteriology laboratory varied to a staggering degree. In one year, five doctors sent in 62 per cent of the throat swabs, while 40 others submitted none. Such findings — similar reports have been published in the USA — imply that antibiotics are not being administered properly.

Another study, published in 1976, set out to determine how much people other than doctors know about antibiotics. Drs Dianne Chandler and A. E. Dugdale, at Mater Children's Hospital, South Brisbane, asked 103 parents of child patients a series of questions. Fifty five per cent of the parents thought that antibiotics killed viruses (which they do not because viruses are not cells) but only 46 per cent believed that they killed bacteria (which they do). Thirteen per cent opined that antibiotics were merely a stronger form of aspirin and 15 per cent said that penicillin was not an antibiotic. Three-quarters of the parents felt that antibiotics should be given routinely for colds and influenza; 40 per cent opted for them for gastro-enteritis.

National Health Service prescribing statistics in Britain show that antibiotics continue to be used indiscriminately for diarrhoeal illness, without any attempt to diagnose those few cases where such treatment is important; that chloramphenicol is still prescribed for infections (often trivial ones) other than typhoid fever; and that young children and pregnant women receive tetracyclines, despite proof that they can harm the development of a child's bones and teeth. It is not clear who is more to blame for such abuse. Some doctors certainly mislead their patients by suggesting (usually on no evidence whatever) that 'a virus' is to blame for an illness, and then prescribing antibiotics. But patients also demand antibiotics for trivial conditions, and receive them against the better judgement of their practitioners. Nearly half a century after Fleming's observation which led to the introduction of penicillin, it and its successors are being ill used. The result is that these 'wonder drugs' have lost much of their wonder. Their efficacy has been eroded by misapplication to a point where they could, indeed, become no more than historical curiosities in the foreseeable future.

Medicine and mortality

If that were to happen, would we be plunged back into the Dark Ages? Would infectious disease pose a horrendous threat to our well-being? These are ticklish questions, and the only way we can begin to answer them is to examine the evidence of history. A considerable argument rages about the impact of

modern medicine on health, ill health and especially population size. What the advocates of both points of view agree is
that scientific medicine, particularly antimicrobial warfare
founded on specific aetiology, was a considerably lesser force
than might be imagined. Thus immunisation against
diphtheria, introduced on a wide scale around 1940, appears
to have had a dramatic effect on the incidence of the disease.
The number of cases in Britain fell by between fifty and sixty
thousand each year until about 1955, since when there have
been only sporadic outbreaks. However, if we take a longer
time scale over the past century, and alter the criteria, we see a
very different picture. Diphtheria deaths in children went
down continuously from 1,300 per year in 1860 to under 300
per year in 1940, with a particularly sharp drop around 1900
when antitoxin was first used. Yet the steepest decline was
between 1865 and 1875 — before the diphtheria bacillus had
even been isolated.

A graph over the same period covering the commonest
infectious diseases of childhood (scarlet fever, measles, whooping cough and diphtheria) shows the death rate falling
regularly, with only a small inflection at the very end reflecting
the introduction of immunisation and antibiotics. While the
achievements of medical science should not be disregarded,
therefore, the returns secured by vaccines and anti-microbial
drugs need to be put in perspective. Over the long term,
greater prosperity (and thus improved nutrition, sanitation
and hygiene) have been far greater influences on the pattern of
infectious disease than the mounting of chemical warfare on
the microbial world.

Thomas McKeown, who has made a special study of the
effects of modern medicine on the British population, claims
that its contribution to declining mortality was not significant
until the second quarter of this century — by which time the
larger proportion of the total fall had already been achieved.
According to Professor McKeown, the advent of BCG vaccination made little or no difference to the decline of mortality
from tuberculosis in England and Wales. Streptomycin

reduced mortality by about half when it was introduced in 1947, but over the whole period since cause of death was first registered its contribution to the reduction in deaths was about 3 per cent. Similarly, McKeown, finds that the arrival of chemotherapy had a moderate effect on mortality from bacterial pneumonia in the age groups 0 - 14 and 45 - 64, but that the influence on deaths at all ages was small. It was certainly not the main reason for the continued decline of the death rate, which was well established from the beginning of the century.

The conclusion we should draw from such figures is not that vaccines and antibiotics have been of no value, but that their impact on mortality and associated illness has been small compared with other factors. Professor McKeown's work implies that:

... the modern improvement in health was initiated and carried quite a long way with little contribution from science and technology, except for the epidemiological investigations of environmental conditions in the eighteenth and early nineteenth centuries. This was true of the increase in food production, the beginning of hygiene measures and control of numbers. These advances resulted from simple but fundamental observations on everyday life: conservation of fertility increased agricultural output, hygiene measures prevented infectious diseases, and limitation of the number of births improved the conditions of life for parents and their children.

Infectious disease was not a major problem for early man. Neither is it today for wild animals. Smaller, more widely spaced families, a sparser population and better nutrition appear to be the three main reasons why the hunter-gatherers enjoyed comparative freedom from infection. They had no need of magic bullets. But all that changed with the appearance of agricultural civilisations and, later, industrialisation.

Habit and heart disease

In April 1976 a working party of the Royal College of Physicians and the British Cardiac Society published a report entitled *Prevention of Coronary Heart Disease*. It was the product of one of the most comprehensive of several recent studies, on both sides of the Atlantic, intended to throw light on a condition that is now the major cause of death in middle and old age in the developed countries. Cardiovascular disease — disease of the heart and blood vessels — has indeed been termed a 'disease of civilisation': it seems to have been relatively uncommon among the hunter-gatherers but has increased viciously with industrialisation. What is striking about the 1976 report and others like it is that they owe nothing to the concept of specific aetiology. They all cover the familiar ground of lifestyle, smoking, blood pressure, fats in the bloodstream, obesity, physical activity, stress, and many other factors which are thought to influence the occurrence of heart attacks. But there is never a hint of specific cause or specific cure.

What we do know is that cardiovascular disease follows from two changes that accompany ageing: rising blood pressure (hypertension) and degeneration of the walls of the arteries (atherosclerosis). Substantial deterioration in both increases the likelihood of both heart attacks and strokes. This combination is relatively common in US Negroes. Atherosclerosis by itself is more clearly associated with a heightened risk of heart attacks, as in American Whites, while high blood pressure without atherosclerosis is characterised by a greater incidence of strokes, but not of heart attacks (as in Japan).

The marked rise in death rates from coronary disease in recent decades in many industrial countries is also unquestionable. But all of the many strenuous attempts to pinpoint discrete causes have failed or at best yielded ambiguous results. The joint working party at the Royal College of Physicians and British Cardiac Society does no more than identify 'risk factors' — and cloud the issue even further by admitting that 'factor' implies a more explicit degree of causation than we really know to exist. 'Risk indicators', they suggest, might be a better term.

A family history of heart trouble is a significant indicator, as is smoking. Sedentary habits, and perhaps a stressful occupation, may also play their part. The danger is greater for those with two or more risk factors. The man with a high concentration of fats in his bloodstream, whose parents and grandparents died in early middle age of heart attacks, who smokes heavily and takes little exercise, has demonstrably more chance of succumbing than a non-smoking daily jogger with low blood fats and no hereditary predisposition. But in none of this is there anything resembling specific aetiology. All is a balance of probabilities.

The working party was particularly concerned about diet. Population studies throughout the world have identified a strong positive relationship between the average amount of cholesterol in the bloodstream and the incidence of coronary heart disease in a community. Moreover, the cholesterol level correlates with the percentage of total calories derived from what chemists call saturated (mostly animal rather than vegetable) fats in the diet. So the report recommends that people should reduce their intake of saturated fats, and substitute polyunsaturated vegetable fats. Such advice has been widely publicised in most developed countries in recent years, and is assiduously followed by many of those anxious to minimise their chances of suffering a heart attack.

But even this idea remains contentious, despite the vast amount of research behind it. In July following the 1976 report, the Department of Health circulated all doctors in the UK with the working party's conclusions, thereby officially endorsing them. Shortly afterwards, one of the country's most distinguished physicians, Sir John McMichael, wrote to *The Lancet* to complain. He felt that the report was based on narrow epidemiological studies and neglected other work conflicting with some of its recommendations. Thus direct examination of coronary arteries in living persons (by the

X-ray technique known as angiography) has shown there to be no difference between those with high and average fat levels in the bloodstream; one report indicated that no combination of three factors (smoking, hypertension and cholesterol) had any influence on the appearance of the arteries. The use of drugs which diminish greatly the amount of circulating cholesterol has proved insignificant in reducing the risk of coronary mortality. And, most frustratingly, there is puzzling evidence about the high death rate from heart attacks among Finnish lumberjacks, who consume a diet exceedingly rich in animal fat. Sir John McMichael cites one diligent study showing that the higher coronary mortality in east Finland was due to the strenuous work of the lumberjacks and not to their raised cholesterol levels—which were equally high in west Finland, where the corresponding death rate was 50 per cent lower. 'It is better to trust to luck than to foster neurosis by pretence that we can save lives by interfering with life habits,' he concluded. 'Much of the advice is good general advice, but coronary disability and mortality are unlikely to be changed.'

Specific aetiology has failed to account for coronary heart disease or for its increase with industrialisation. It is conceivable that the problem is simply highly intractable and that a discrete cause of this modern malady will come to light in the future. All the evidence suggests otherwise. What that evidence has done, for all its inadequacy, is to turn attention away from specific determinants, towards behaviour and lifestyle as areas where the answers must surely be found.

Health and smoking

One element of lifestyle, smoking, appears in a rapidly worsening light as an adverse influence on a range of different diseases. The World Health Organisation, reviewing the growing dossier on the habit, concludes that smoking is 'one of the greatest avoidable health hazards of modern times'. Epidemiological evidence from many countries, the WHO claims, implicates tobacco smoking as a causative factor in coronary heart disease, chronic bronchitis, lung cancer, duodenal ulcer, abortion, stillbirth and neonatal death, and cancers of the tongue, larynx, oesophagus, pancreas and bladder. One large survey, begun in Japan in 1967, had shown by 1975 that mortality was 22 per cent higher among cigarette smokers, both male and female, than among non-smokers.

The failure of specific aetiology is exemplified by the continued controversy as to whether smoking causes lung cancer. There is a transparently clear association between the two. Moreover, the greater the number of cigarettes smoked, the more likely the smoker is to develop carcinoma of the lung. Together with evidence that deaths from lung cancer have increased around the world as cigarette smoking has become a common habit, these facts have persuaded most experts that the relationship is a causal one. Such was the case mounted originally in Britain by Dr Richard Doll and Dr Austin Bradford Hill in the 1950s, which has led to official action to dissuade people from smoking. But objections were raised, notably by the psychologist Dr Hans Eysenck and more recently by the medical physicist Professor Philip Burch. Though arguing from different premises, each pointed out the possibility of a different explanation for the observed relationship. The propensity to smoke and the propensity to develop lung cancer may each derive from some other, inbred factor.

Over the years, much more evidence has been garnered and some of the original doubters have been converted by data showing that, by giving up the habit, smokers can apparently improve their chances of not contracting lung cancer. Yet the charge is still not fully proven. Nor can the truth be established conclusively without the impossible: a planned experiment with randomly selected groups of people who are divided into two groups and asked to smoke or not smoke during a trial period. For many of us, the likelihood of a causal link between smoking and lung cancer is a strong deterrent, even without definitive proof. Besides, the overall medical evidence against smoking is impressive; the indictment does not rest on lung cancer alone. Nonetheless, it has to be admitted that a weak point remains in the now orthodox position. Many people smoke heavily and do not succumb to lung cancer. There could be no more spectacular failure of the theory of specific aetiology.

Cancer—no magic secret

'Search for *the* cause may be a hopeless pursuit because most disease states are the indirect outcome of a constellation of circumstances rather than the direct result of single determinant factors,' writes René Dubos. His comments apply forcibly to cancers. True, several chemicals, as well as forms of radiation, have been incriminated in the production of malignancy. Twenty such carcinogens, for example, have come to light in industry and in use as drugs. They include ultraviolet light as a cause of skin cancer in farmers and sailors, asbestos as an agent of tumours in the membranes surrounding the lungs, and the drug chlornaphazene as the cause of cancer of the pelvis. But we should take care to use the words 'cause' and 'agent' cautiously here. While the incriminating evidence was strong in these cases, and appropriate action was rightly taken to prevent further exposure, such substances are mostly weak carcinogens. Disease is usually produced only after prolonged, intensive exposure. Some of those exposed do not contract the disease. And in no case do we understand how the agent acts against the cells of the body. As Dubos suggests, there may well be no single 'secret of cancer'. The term 'cancer' could prove to be more an adjective than a noun, a descriptive word we have applied to a large number of conditions which have certain features in common.

One of the most stimulating recent ideas about the origin of cancers has emerged not from orthodox laboratory research, but from investigations into food consumption in Africa and elsewhere by Dr Denis Burkitt. He believes that the Western diet, with its relative deficiency in fibre and high proportion of meat, fat and refined carbohydrates, may play a role in the production of malignancy. Burkitt bases his thesis on observations that several diseases, including appendicitis and diverticulitis as well as cancers, are common in developed countries but rare in rural Africa. Corresponding with this is the contrast between the Western low-residue diet and that of rural Africa with its large content of fibre. High-residue food passes more quickly through the intestines, and this may be significant in relation to cancer. Burkitt's hypothesis is still a hypothesis. But his style of investigation seems to offer a more hopeful avenue for further research than repeated laboratory attempts to discover *the* cause of the disease.

When the Society for Social Responsibility in Science, in Australia, published its recent book *The Magic Bullet* on the limitations of modern medicine, the following quotation was used as the introduction:

> The magic substance is invaluable to the medical profession . . . In the case of cancer it cures by touch. Stranger still, it touches without direct contact. Nothing is observed to happen when radium is brought close to the cancerous growth. But a few days later the growth begins to shrivel; eventually it disappears without a scar, and terrible disfigured parts become normal.

Such enthusiasm for a magic bullet to vanquish cancer (from *The Children's New Illustrated Encyclopaedia*, 1946) was, alas, premature. Many extensive programmes have been mounted to synthesise and test chemicals to deploy against different tumours — on essentially the same basis that Paul Ehrlich experimented with arsenical compounds for syphilis. One of the most massive efforts of this sort was at the National Cancer Institute, Bethesda, in the USA. Such projects have yielded a few cytotoxic drugs — substances which do preferentially more damage to rapidly dividing tumour cells than to normal tissue. But the returns have been puny in relation to the expenditure. Cancer therapy has made disappointingly little progress.

Statistics of survival

Just how bleak the picture really is can be seen from figures
compiled by the American journalist Dan Greenberg and published in 1975 in the *Columbia Journalism Review*. The
starting-point was a statement by Dr Frank Rauscher, director
of the National Cancer Institute, that 'the five year survival
rate for cancer patients in the 1930s was about one in five.
Today the figure is one in three.' As Greenberg showed,
however, closer inspection of the official figures confirmed
that most of the improvement since the 1930s was achieved
before 1955. Over the past two decades survival rates have not
altered much, and some have even deteriorated. Thus the
chances of surviving one year with cancer of the colon in the
USA fell from 68 per cent in 1965-69 to 65 per cent in
1970-71. The five-year survival rate for cervical cancer rose
from 47 per cent in 1941-49 to 59 per cent in 1951-59, but
then dropped to 56 per cent in the period 1965-69. Five-year
survival rates for cancer of the stomach and rectum have
remained at around 12 and 40 per cent respectively since 1950.
For oesophageal cancer the figure declined from 4 to 3 per
cent over the twenty-five years up to 1975. What seems to have
happened during the 1940s and early 1950s is not that more
people were surviving cancer. A greater number were with-
standing cancer *surgery*. Antibiotics and blood transfusion
had reduced the toll of life from such operations. But since
1955, when deaths from surgery became negligible, the prospect of surviving most common cancers has changed little.

   The National Cancer Institute figures show that for a range
of cancers accounting for 78 per cent of the total incidence of
the disease the upwards trend in survival rates has not
exceeded a few percentage points. And for some tumours
(representing about 13 per cent of incidence) the rate has
fallen. Though improvements of five or more per cent in
survival rates have been achieved for the remaining 22 per cent
of cases, the overall picture is far gloomier than that conveyed
by the cancer research organisations. Moreover, even these

figures probably give an unjustly favourable impression. Cure rates may be lower than reported, because 'false positives', such as undiagnosed lesions that later turn out to be non-malignant, are included in the statistics.

Meanwhile, as other conditions have been progressively eliminated, cancer has become correspondingly more important as a fatal disease (particularly among children). Fifty years ago cancer was the certified cause of one death in every nine in Great Britain; today the figure is one in five. A decrease in the incidence of some tumours has been more than compensated for by an increase in others. Sir Richard Doll calculates that, in the absence of other causes of death, a third of all men and a quarter of women will develop cancer before the age of 75 — slightly less than the age which half the population now achieves. 'Cancer was never just a disease of the old, but its treatment and prevention have now become a matter of serious concern for the young and middle-aged,' Sir Richard concludes. As we shall see in Chapter 7 prevention, not treatment, seems the main hope for the future. Despite astronomical expenditure, most research oriented towards specific therapy has not paid off. The US National Cancer Institute's budget for 1975 was 669 million dollars — compared with 303 million dollars allocated to the National Heart Institute. Between 1970 and 1975 (following political battles over cancer funding between President Nixon and Senator Edward Kennedy) appropriations for the institute rose by 280 per cent. Heart research received a 104 per cent increase and all other research at the National Institutes of Health an extra 11 per cent. The vastly greater proportion of the cancer research money went into investigations designed to reveal the specific causes of cancer or to fabricate specific therapy. Yet in 1975 cancer deaths in the USA increased by 7 per cent — compared with an average annual rise of around one per cent over the previous decade.

Specific aetiology—a bad influence?

So far in this chapter we have been examining the deficiencies of specific aetiology as an explanatory tool. But there is another type of criticism which must be laid at the door of the theory: it has encouraged an unsatisfactory degree of specialisation in medicine, unnecessary prescribing, and a tendency to believe that all manner of non-diseases are pathological entities. The urge to specify has had consequences which have been bad for medicine, bad for patients, and bad for society.

Consider, for example, the following two authentic case histories, condensed from reports by William St Clair Symmers.

A gynaecologist removed an ovarian cyst from a young woman. The tumour was moderate in size and on the right side. It had come to light first when the woman consulted her doctor because of occasional attacks of vague pain in her lower abdomen, mainly on the right. She was chesty after the operation, and coughing caused her considerable pain in the region of the wound. On the fifth morning her temperature rose, her pulse was racing, and her blood contained abnormal numbers of white cells. These were sure signs of infection. Her abdomen was distended and there was tenderness, particularly on the lower right. Suspecting a complication of the operation, the gynaecologist reopened her abdomen. He discovered early peritonitis from a perforated appendix, which was gangrenous. He sent for a general surgeon who took over and removed the appendix. The patient convalesced without further trouble.

The staggering part of this story comes in an admission afterwards by the gynaecologist. During the first operation he had noticed that the woman's appendix was unhealthy. It was covered in fibrous tissue and probably contained a faecolith — a stone-like body made of compacted faeces. But he did not take out the appendix 'because he considered it wrong to meddle in the province of general surgery'.

A second example also concerns a gynaecologist and a

general surgeon. The gynaecologist was examining a young housewife who had been admitted to hospital for investigation of her irregular periods. During the examination, she collapsed with vomiting and sudden, severe abdominal pain. Over a year earlier she had been treated for a duodenal ulcer, and when she collapsed the gynaecologist assumed that the ulcer had perforated. So he called for a general surgeon, who agreed to operate. What he found was an abdomen full of blood from a ruptured tubal pregnancy (in a fallopian tube). He immediately sent for the gynaecologist, who meanwhile had left for another hospital but returned and, within twenty minutes of his colleague's call for help, had stopped the bleeding and removed the tube.

What is appalling about this second incident is that, while awaiting the specialist, the general surgeon had held a swab against the bleeding area in a not very effective attempt to control the loss of blood. The delay in dealing with the emergency nearly cost the patient her life, as she was bleeding much more than the surgeon realised and had lost nearly all of her blood. The general surgeon explained afterwards that he had not dealt with the tubal rupture because, although he was familiar with the procedure, and had assisted at such operations while a student, 'he did not consider it right to meddle in the province of a specialty'.

Such incidents, reflecting extreme consequences of medical specialisation, may be infrequent. What is by no means unusual is for hospital patients to be dealt with not as whole people but as clinical specimens labelled with particular categories of affliction and treated exclusively by corresponding specialists. They may be cross-referred from one expert to another, each coping skilfully with the pathology of a precise region of the body. Between them the patient is easily made to feel more like an anatomical or metabolic exhibit than a real person.

A division of specialised care between the different disciplines of medicine — surgery, with its sub-specialists; obstetrics and gynaecology; endocrinology; rheumatology; and the rest — is inevitable if the various experts are going to become adequately skilled in their own fields. But there is no reason why the patient should be the loser. All too often, he or she is forgotten amidst the specialisms of high technology.

Such a failing is most common in teaching hospitals, with their combination of frontier science and an obligation to teach specialised medicine to young doctors. The situation was admirably summed up in an exchange between two British consultants, the neurologist Dr Henry Miller and the psychiatrist Dr Hugh Freeman, during a debate held in 1972. Freeman declared: 'A great deal of highly sophisticated medicine completely ignores the emotional and psychological effects of the procedures used on the patient. Many patients who go through the very complex procedures of teaching hospitals come out desperately frightened and uncertain of what has been going on.' To which Miller replied: '. . and cured! Let's get one fact right. Where it is possible to measure the results of treatment — in routine surgery, for example — the advantages of being treated in a teaching rather than a non-teaching hospital are impeccably validated by epidemiology and statistics.'

Here the robust approach by Henry Miller, confident of the value of science-based medicine, of specific therapies efficiently administered, contrasts starkly with the wider concern of Hugh Freeman that patients are indeed treated like specimens in certain hospitals. Some of those patients will themselves be sufficiently robust in mind and body scarcely to notice. Others will certainly suffer as a result.

For some, alas, the categories and specialties are irrelevant. That was clear from a courageous article, printed in the *Guardian* in January 1977, written by Mrs Meg Murray, who was arguing the case for euthanasia. Over forty years earlier Mrs Murray had developed multiple sclerosis, but the disease had occurred only as occasional acute attacks, none lasting more than a week. 'Now the pattern of disease has changed, it has become progressive,' wrote Mrs Murray. 'My muscles are gradually failing and this failure is complicated by arthritis.

It was suggested to me by a rheumatologist that I went into hospital to try to decide which [of the two maladies] was doing what. But I declined. What's in a name?'

The misuse of pharmacy

Unnecessary drug consumption is another consequence of specific aetiology. Many of the conditions for which we purchase panaceas across the counter are imaginary. They include 'night starvation', 'tired blood', and similar epithets much exploited by the patent medicine industry. Doctors also compose many prescriptions, often for genuinely potent medicines, largely to authenticate by specific nomenclature their patients' real or imaginary illnesses. Richard Asher has claimed, on the basis of considerable experience, that 90 per cent of the bottles of medicine dispensed for coughs could be replaced, without any change in efficacy, by 'portentously flavoured fluid'. Most cough mixtures depend on the action of expectorants — substances that promote the coughing up of sputum. But expectorants have no effect unless they are given in doses nearly strong enough to cause vomiting. Similarly, large volumes of 'tonics' are still prescribed, though there is no pharmacological evidence that they have any value whatever.

So too with mass consumption of vitamin preparations — surely the most absurd consequence of a profound belief in the efficacy of chemical cures. As we saw in Chapter 3, vitamins are unquestionably beneficial to people living on a grossly deficient diet. However, the amount and variety of food consumed daily in the developed West contains more than enough of all the necessary vitamins. There is little to justify their wholesale consumption in these countries — other than the all too prevalent belief that a drug cure exists for everything. In a characteristically honest passage, Dr Asher writes:

Many of us give nicotinic acid to anyone with a sore tongue. Probably not one in 100 of those so treated receives any benefit because not one in 100 of them has pellagra. Nicotinic acid cures the sore tongue of pellagra but does not cure all sore tongues, just as quinine will cure the rigors of malaria but does not stop all rigors. The other vitamins are used equally irrationally, and because rats fed on a vitamin E deficient diet have miscarriages, vast quantities of vitamin E are doled out to barren women all over the world, with no benefit to them.

A typical example of misguided therapy is hormone replacement for women, the purpose of which is to combat the unpleasantness of the menopause. Several drugs have been introduced for this purpose since 1974. All contain some form of oestrogen, the female hormone secreted by the ovaries which plays a central role in sustaining the activity of the reproductive organs, including the vagina, uterus and breasts, as well as being responsible for many of the secondary attributes of femininity. At the change of life, the body's production of oestrogen falls to a low level. So an obvious possibility is to counter the adverse effects of the menopause by administering this hormone as a drug. A new clinic, run by the Association of Women's Health Care, opened in London in 1977 with that specific intent.

The defect in this approach is that the menopause is a natural phenomenon, and one which should not be—indeed cannot be—neutralised by consumption of a specific chemical. Women who have been persuaded that hormone replacement therapy, given from middle age onwards, is an elixir of youth must be doomed to disappointment. True, there are occasional menopausal complications, particularly a thinning of the lining of the vagina (making intercourse painful), which can be relieved by oestrogens. But tablets cannot turn the clock back.

'Is grief an illness?' was the headline of a recent editorial in *The Lancet* which explored another situation in which recourse to chemotherapy is now routine. Before the rise of scientific medicine, bereavement was followed naturally by a period of mourning. The bereaved were helped by their friends and relatives and by their own inner resources. Today, a doctor is more than likely to prescribe a tranquilliser, sedative or sleeping pill to 'treat' the condition. For many people nowadays the consolations of religion are no longer meaningful, so it may not be surprising that solace is sought in chemical panaceas. *The Lancet* drew attention to one survey of forty-six bereaved relatives in a Glasgow general practice, in which three-quarters of the smokers and nearly a third of the alcohol drinkers increased their consumption. 'It might be better', *The Lancet* concluded, 'if pharmacologically less harmful drugs such as the benzodiazepines [drugs of the Librium/Valium group] either were more liberally supplied by doctors or were even available over the counter at pharmacies.'

The medicalisation of problems

Bereavement and the menopause are two examples of personal problems that are being 'medicalised'. The Office of Health Economics, a UK body financed by the pharmaceutical industry, has drawn attention to a parallel medicalisation of social troubles, such that doctors are being required to deal with matters beyond their expertise and training: 'Many now act as advisers, comforters, and father confessors on a wide range of matters which would never previously have been regarded as medical problems. These include, for example, family strife, financial difficulties, dissatisfaction or insecurity at work, sexual problems and deviant behaviour such as alcoholism, violence or even straightforward crime.' One wonders what proportion of such problems are dealt with by genuine counselling, and what proportion are dismissed with a prescription for the appropriate chemical. Drug advertisements certainly point the way: 'Loss of life style ... sweet marital bliss has turned sour, and everything seems beyond her capabilities ... Sinequan could help her cope.' 'I was so wretched I burst into tears ... I felt so irritable. It wasn't as if he'd shouted at me.

He only asked me to iron his blue shirt, but at that moment, anything was too much for me . . . In a moment of emotional crisis . . . Tofranil Geigy.' One potion is promoted to doctors in Britain as 'the workers' antidepressant.' In 1977 an estimated 25 million prescriptions were dispensed in Britain for tranquillisers.

One attempt to find out more about this mass medication has been reported by Professor W. H. Trethowan. He found that of the 255.9 million family doctor prescriptions dispensed in England in 1972 those for medicines acting on the central nervous system formed easily the largest proportion. The greater part of these — 17.7 per cent of the total — were for drugs of the type given to treat psychiatric disorder. Having looked into the reasons why they were prescribed, Professor Trethowan concludes that such drugs are probably being used increasingly to try to modify personal and interpersonal processes. 'One of several dangers inherent in this is the promotion of what may be regarded as a positive feedback mechanism', he points out. 'The more the habit of prescribing pills for personal problems grows among doctors, the more it is likely that their patients may come increasingly to demand this kind of solution to their difficulties — a solution that is likely to turn out to be a non-solution.'

Antidote or correction?

Like the abuse of antibiotics, recourse to medication to relieve emotional and social troubles stems from an antidotal, rather than a corrective, approach to biological maladjustments which manifest themselves as disease, or are so named. The right and in the long term more effective way to combat the ravages of salmonellosis in calves is by keeping the animals in cleaner, less oppressive conditions, not by deploying specific antimicrobial drugs indiscriminately. The sound way to cope with anxiety or depression is by tackling their root causes rather than by clouding brain function with tranquillisers.

Dispensing pills is invariably the easier solution, but sooner or later it is self-defeating.

Yet antidotal medicine, based on glamorous technology and magic bullets, continues to consume by far the largest slice of our resources for health care. One example will suffice. In both the USA and Britain, the major effort in coping with cardiovascular disease in recent years has gone into improving hospital facilities for treating victims of heart attacks. The main sign of this has been the setting up of highly complex and costly intensive care units — of which 3,000 had been created in American hospitals by the end of 1971. And this has been done without any convincing proof of their efficacy. Several reports have compared the results of treatment at home, in a hospital ward, and in an intensive care unit, without showing more than marginal advantages for the infinitely more expensive arrangements. One difficulty is that about half of all coronary deaths occur within two hours of the attack — which, allowing for delays in summoning a doctor and reaching hospital, means that such cases are beyond the possible reach of the most sophisticated treatment. Moreover, a person who has suffered one heart attack has a greatly increased chance of having another. These and other factors conspire to thwart intensive care of much of its theoretical value — so the cost of such facilities becomes disproportionately large.

Thus the failures (and there have, of course, been successes) of the machine approach to man, and of the specific therapy of disease, have important financial and political consequences. Medical determinism has not only distorted our judgements in medical research and medical care. It has also wielded undue influence in determining our use of resources.

5
Mind over matter

As a schoolboy, I professed vague ill health occasionally on days when exceptionally horrid lessons or masters were on the timetable. Gastric symptoms sometimes appeared as evident proof. When the family doctor was consulted, he never found anything, though once or twice he obliged by pronouncing that the boy had 'gastritis' or 'a chill'. An appropriate bottle of innocuous liquid would accompany his diagnosis, and everyone then felt that the malady had been authenticated.

Specific aetiology has nothing to say about this sort of thing. It does not illuminate the problems of alcoholism or asthma or insomnia or that mysterious affliction, anorexia nervosa, in which the victim rejects more and more food items, believing them to be harmful, and which leads to progressive emaciation. It sheds no light on the recovery from serious illness that occasionally follows a visit to Lourdes or treatment by a faith healer. Specific aetiology is irrelevant to most everyday problems seen by doctors. The theory which has formed the main axis of medical thought for the past century is of little use in probing some of the commonest and most human aspects of ill health. Its most conspicuous influence is often to ensure that the doctor, consciously or unconsciously, places a specific label — anxiety neurosis, neurasthenia, virus infection — on what is not a mechanical or metabolic fault but is more accurately described as a state. The condition may be frustration, worry, thwarted ambition, boredom — dis*ease* rather than discrete disease. In describing such dis*ease* we are no more skilled than was Hippocrates with his picture of imbalance in the bodily humours. Worse. Today's doctors are less likely to discern real troubles. The modern habit of thought is to diagnose medical rather than personal or social grounds for ill health. So root causes are ignored, tensions and fears are suppressed by medication.

The riddle of colitis

There are, of course, distinct diseases which orthodox medicine has labelled 'psychosomatic'. Ulcerative colitis, the scaly skin disease psoriasis, and peptic and duodenal ulcers are examples of conditions with clear physical symptoms but in which psychology and personality appear to play an important role. The inability of specific aetiology to explain or even clarify that role is particularly striking with ulcerative colitis — inflammation of the colon. Dysentery produces an acute form of colitis, and here the exact cause can be securely identified: the bacterium *Shigella dysenteriae*. But for practical purposes in developed countries colitis means a chronic complaint, of which there are two forms: ulcerative colitis, and the less severe mucous colitis. Psychological factors are thought to be active in triggering off both conditions. How (and indeed whether) this happens, remains a mystery.

Ulcerative colitis has been studied most intensively, yielding a vast literature of clinical reports, research papers, and surveys. Dr D. C. Murray pioneered the field, with a psychological investigation of twelve patients in 1930. He discovered 'a well-marked time-relationship between the outbreak of an emotional disturbance and the onset of symptoms'. The commonest source of anxiety was mental conflict concerned with marriage, and Dr Murray concluded that the patients had faced their problems in an 'inadequate and juvenile manner'. A little later, Dr E. Wittkower conducted personality studies on forty unselected patients with ulcerative colitis and found that before the onset of disease most of them had had psychological abnormalities and disorders well beyond the range of individual differences in the population at large. There was 'a clear-cut emotional trauma, serious enough to be regarded as a precipitating agent' immediately before the appearance of colitis in twenty-eight of the patients.

During the 1950s Dr G. L. Engel in the USA reviewed this evidence and much more, scrutinising the records of 39 of his own patients and published reports on a further 700, written by many other practitioners. Four factors emerged with impressive consistency. These were defects in personality long preceding the colitis, dependent and restricted relationships with other people, psychopathology in the mothers, and failure to achieve full heterosexual development. At about the same time Dr L. Krasner carried out an intensive survey using intelligence and personality tests designed to provide more objective evidence than that gained from other investigators' somewhat anecdotal studies. He compared victims of duodenal ulcer or ulcerative colitis with patients who had never contracted these or any other conditions considered to be psychosomatic. The results confirmed earlier descriptions of colitis patients as passive, insecure, shy, sensitive, and moody. This group also did best in the intelligence test.

Some medical practitioners have been so impressed by such data that they have relied on psychotherapy as the mainstay of treatment. Others have favoured physical solutions: drugs and diet. Antibiotics have been administered in a half-hearted belief that bacteria might be involved. Yet comparison of the two styles of therapy reveal no clear differences. In a famous study, Dr W. J. Grace and his colleagues managed one set of thirty-four patients largely by psychotherapy aimed at relieving stress, and a matched group by physical treatment. The first group fared better—but only marginally so.

There are, moreover, rigorous investigations which have revealed no psychological basis whatever to ulcerative colitis. One of the most telling, carried out by Dr F. Feldman and colleagues, was published in 1967. A psychological comparison of thirty-four patients with the general population and with patients admitted to hospital for other intestinal conditions showed that the great majority of colitis victims were 'normal' with regard to personality and psychiatric illness. Only a small minority had experienced an emotional shock or trauma shortly before their illness began. Seven of the patients had received psychotherapy. This had helped three of them to cope with their colitis, but in none did the treatment seem to have influenced the disease's progress.

If further negative evidence is required, it comes from a survey by Drs E. D. Acheson and M. D. Nefzger of ulcerative colitis among men in the US Army. Every patient was matched with a corresponding non-sufferer of the same age, sex, and rank, but the comparison revealed no differences in military conduct, intelligence, educational attainments, or income before enlistment. A similar comparative study by Dr M. Monk in Baltimore revealed no variations in educational achievements, amount of life lived with parents or alone, degree of social contact with others before the onset of the illness, or the number of bereavements or marital disagreements in the month preceding the symptoms of colitis. Dr Monk's research was aimed specifically at uncovering differences in social environment between patients with ulcerative colitis and the population from which they came. The one significant finding was that the colitis victims were more likely to have had fathers who had died during their childhood. This correlates with the opinion of another investigator, Dr J. W. Paulley, that 'the disease is associated with a well-defined personality not uncommonly related to the unfortunate effect of overpossessive mothers'.

Taking all of this and other evidence as a piece, it seems incontrovertible that personality and emotional experiences are relevant to the onset of chronic colitis. Despite the negative reports, there are too many positive claims—and correlations between them—for the idea to be dismissed as an illusion. Perhaps more informative than meticulous surveys with personality questionnaires are the clinical observations of experienced practitioners, which have also strengthened the psychosomatic theory of the disease. Subjective impressions, gained by careful person-to-person diagnosis in the Hippocratic tradition, may be far more meaningful than detailed scientific analysis in throwing light on a condition of this sort. The conflict of hard evidence about ulcerative colitis which has emerged so far illustrates above all the bluntness of the tools with which we have tried to examine the disease.

Mind over matter

If that is true of a condition strongly suspected of being 'psychosomatic', it must apply even more strongly to diseases known to have a physical aetiology but which from time to time behave so perversely as to imply that they have a psychological component. What, for example, of the genuine illness — perhaps a gastric upset or a respiratory infection with an incontestable runny nose — which arrives as soon as one relaxes after an exhausting period of work? What of the genuine symptoms that can appear in the opposite situation, just before a hateful confrontation or unwelcome business trip?

The Medical Research Council in Britain has begun spending a little money in exploring such questions, and some of the first results were reported in 1976. One investigation has been carried out at the Common Cold Research Unit, Salisbury, by Dr Sylvia Reed and Dr Wallace Craig, working with Dr Richard Totman, a psychologist from Nuffield College, Oxford. In scrupulously controlled tests, forty-eight volunteers at the unit were inoculated with common cold viruses. Half were then confronted with a choice of taking a new 'drug' (actually an inactive placebo), but were told that afterwards their stomach juices would have to be examined via a stomach tube. The other half were neither offered the drug nor warned about the use of a stomach tube. As a result, the cold symptoms in the first group (as assessed by an independent clinician) were more severe than those in the untreated group. The likely explanation is that the anxiety generated as a result of taking a difficult decision had a real effect on the course of the volunteers' respiratory illness.

'Explanation' here is, of course, a misnomer. Using the word psychosomatic no more explains this mysterious finding than it accounts for the equally puzzling but well authenticated report by Dr Henry Beecher in 1959 that 35 out of 100 surgical patients experienced genuine relief from pain after receiving an ineffective placebo when they were expecting morphine. Again, is the word 'ineffective' appropriate? The patients' anticipation that they were to be given morphine was sufficient to relieve their discomfort. So was the placebo active or not? We can certainly say that it was not physically effective in interfering, according to the dictates of specific aetiology, with cells of the nervous system. Yet the end result was as positive as would have followed from administration of the expected morphine.

Dr J. A. Maga has discovered a quirk of human sensitivity just as remarkable and very precise: our expectation of the way something ought to taste affects its real taste. Working at Colorado State University, he found that the colouring of dilute solutions of bitter, sweet, and other substances alters a person's perceptions of their taste. The materials he used were sugar, citric acid, caffeine, and salt. Each was made up in colourless form and also with (tasteless) red, green, or yellow colouring agents added. Young men and women were then asked to sample the liquids from each series, beginning with the most dilute, and to record the point at which they first experienced the particular taste.

The results were surprising. Most of the coloured solutions needed to be more concentrated than the corresponding colourless versions before the subjects were capable of identifying the specific taste — especially sour and bitter. Particular colours had particular effects, suggesting a psychological association of food colours with taste. Green, for example, increased the threshold at which the sweet solution could be tasted. Conversely, yellow colour decreased taste sensitivity. There were several other relationships between (presumably) expectations stemming from the colour associations of particular foods and real ability to experience taste. The only exception was saltiness. Apparently we do not relate saltiness to any colour; none of the coloured salty solutions were detected at significantly different concentrations from the colourless control.

Such findings are impossible to explain on the basis of the picture of the nervous system as first described by Johannes Müller (p.24) and extended by modern research. That plan, showing the various sense organs each receiving and transmitting to the brain specific categories of signal, is doubtless a considerable oversimplification.

Healing by faith?

Unexpected recovery from serious affliction, especially when associated with religious belief or with the powerful personality of a 'faith healer' or the like, is an embarrassment to most members of the medical profession. Firmly wedded to the cause-and-effect relationship enshrined in specific aetiology, they do not relish being asked to 'explain' such incidents. Yet an uncomfortable number of these cures are on the record in medical journals. From time to time books have been published describing them more fully and in a more personal style than is possible in a formal research report. The very purpose of a scientific paper is to set out 'the facts' objectively, purged of all the investigator's feelings and beliefs. No less an authority than Sir Peter Medawar has argued on these grounds that the scientific paper can be considered a fraud, because it pretends to an unrealistic extreme of objectivity in which the research worker imagines that he had no preconceived ideas about the outcome of his work and processed the results by mindless induction.

This explains why personal testimonies are usually more satisfying than bare clinical reports in conveying a full picture of the circumstances surrounding 'miraculous' or extraordinary recovery from dangerous illness. Two such accounts are Dr Christopher Woodard's *A Doctor Heals by Faith* and

Dr Michael Agnellet's *I Accept These Facts*. The first is by a specialist in the undeniably materialistic field of sports injuries, and centres on the time when his two-year-old son regained full health after suffering fulminating meningitis, an infection which seemed destined to prove fatal. Orthodox medical opinion was certainly that the child would die. While acknowledging the importance of medical therapy, Dr Woodard attributed his son's recovery to the faith and prayers of the parents and hundreds of friends. Later he studied 'divine healing' and wrote of further cases in which faith brought about a cure. 'I have a complete conviction', he says, 'that there is no such thing as an incurable disease — no such thing as an easy or difficult case of healing in Christ's name.'

Dr Agnellet is an atheist and materialist who set out to determine the truth about allegedly miraculous cures at Lourdes. He examined the records in the Medical Bureau there, and went back to original sources where possible, finding a series of examples of recovery from cancer and other serious illness that he believes are beyond description by scientific medicine. The book carries a foreward by Dr E. B. Strauss, a physician for psychological medicine at St Bartholomew's Hospital, London, who writes:

> It is inevitable that the author should end with a 'giant question mark', but he will doubtless feel his purpose completely fulfilled if his readers come to believe with him that Lourdes is quite certainly the scene of some remarkable cures, cures moreover that cannot be explained scientifically, and which can only be satisfactorily denied on the improbable basis that there exists a gigantic conspiracy, or the most terrible inefficiency and slovenly investigating by a very reputable body of men.

Apart from exasperation and irritation, orthodox medicine has two replies to challenges about inexplicable healing. The first is to categorise it. When an advanced tumour recedes and a mortally ill patient regains full health, this is known as a 'spontaneous remission'. Again, such terminology does not explain anything. It serves only to place an awkward fact into a specific department and thus remove it from the untidy residue of the unexplained. The second response is marginally more constructive. This is to dismiss the convictions a patient or his family have in the role of faith, prayer, or belief, by insisting that somehow the full resources of the ill person have been mobilised in the fight against disease. The 'will to live', such critics concede under pressure, can help a patient *in extremis*. But they are invariably unenthusiastic about making too much of this, and easily slip back into a trivialisation of the event by using the phrase 'spontaneous recovery'.

Laughter, the best medicine?

A small proportion of medical practitioners are less assured. One such was the medical attendant of Norman Cousins, editor of the *Saturday Review*, whose account of his experiences with a hideous illness is one of the most bizarre medical sagas of recent years. Though the incident occurred in 1964, he did not write about it until 1976, because he was anxious not to raise false hopes among those similarly afflicted. But his recovery had been validated by that time — by any standards — so he felt justified in telling his peculiar story. In August 1964 Cousins flew home to New York with a slight fever following a business trip in the Soviet Union. The malaise, with a general feeling of achiness, increased rapidly. Within a week, Cousins could hardly move his neck, arms, fingers or legs. He entered hospital and his ESR,* which had already shot up to 80, eventually reached 115.

Mr Cousins also began to feel displeased with the hospital — with the routine that suited the convenience of staff rather than patients, with the taking of four different blood samples

*The rate at which red blood cells stick together and sediment in a glass tube. It rises during infections and other conditions.

by four different technicians for four different purposes, with the food, and with the 'surprising lack of respect for basic sanitation'. He complained to his doctor and longstanding friend, Dr William Hitzig, who agreed with the criticisms and did what he could to help. Meanwhile, the illness grew worse. Cousins had great difficulty in moving his limbs and even in turning over in bed. Nodules appeared on his body, and gravel-like substances under the skin. His jaws became almost locked.

Then the diagnosis. After conferring with other experts, Dr Hitzig announced that the verdict was ankylosing spondylitis, a condition in which the collagen in the space between joints is attacked, becoming hardened and calcified. Medical textbooks list it as a 'disease of unknown aetiololgy'. The prognosis appeared grim. One of the experts put the chances of recovery at one in 500; another said he had never witnessed recovery from this comprehensive state.

'All this gave me a great deal to think about,' says Cousins in his account of the affair. 'Up to that time, I had been more or less disposed to let the doctors worry about my condition. But now I felt a compulsion to get into the act. It seemed clear to me that if I was to be that "one case in 500" I had better be something more than a passive observer.' First he began to speculate about the cause of the disease. Dr Hitzig could not be very helpful, but suggested that it might have arisen from heavy metal poisoning or the after-effects of a streptococcal infection. Thinking back to his trip, Cousins remembered that he had slept badly while staying in Moscow because of noise during the night and that on the last day there he caught the exhaust spew of a large jet at point-blank range as it swung around on the tarmac at Moscow airport. Could these events have triggered off the illness?

Rightly or wrongly, Norman Cousins concluded that they may have been significant but that he was probably unduly vulnerable because he was already suffering from 'adrenal exhaustion'. His business trip had been very full and tiring, with many late nights, culminating in a maddening, frustrating last evening caused by various arrangements going awry. Then came the long flight back to the USA on an overcrowded plane. 'By the time we arrived in New York, cleared through the packed customs counters, and got rolling back to Connecticut, I could feel an uneasiness deep in my bones. A week later I was hospitalised.'

Contemplating his condition, Cousins remembered the classic book *The Stress of Life*, in which Hans Seyle showed that emotional tension, such as frustration or suppressed rage, could cause adrenal exhaustion. So what of the possible restorative function of the positive emotions? Was it likely, Cousins asked himself, that 'love, hope, faith, laughter, confidence and the will to live had therapeutic value? Do chemical changes occur only on the downside?' The idea, he deduced, was worth acting upon. First he must inquire about his medication; any drugs likely to be toxic could spoil the plan. Allergy tests showed that he was sensitive to virtually all the medicaments he was receiving — pain-killers and anti-inflammatory agents. But what about the pain if he were to give up these drugs? Cousins felt as though the bones in his spine and practically every joint in his body had been run over by a truck. Nonetheless, he believed that he could tolerate the discomfort if he knew that progress was being made in tackling the basic disease. Then he decided that vitamin C might help to combat the inflammation.

Dr Hitzig listened carefully to these ruminations. He concluded that there was 'nothing undersized about my will to live. He said that what was most important was that I continue to believe in everything I had said. He shared my sense of excitement about the possibilities of my recovery and liked the idea of a partnership.'

So the plan went into effect. Laughter was to be a key component, and a cine projector was acquired along with some film made by Allen Funt, producer of the television programme *Candid Camera*. It worked. 'I made the joyous discovery that 10 minutes of genuine belly laughter had an anaesthetic effect and would give me at least two hours of pain-free sleep. When the pain-killing effect of the laughter wore off, we would switch on the motion-picture projector again, and, not infrequently, it would lead to another pain-free sleep interval.' Sometimes a nurse would read extracts from funny books instead. Before each laughter episode, and several hours afterwards, blood samples were taken for measuring ESR. Each time there was a fall of at least five points. The drop by itself was not substantial, but it held and was cumulative.

There was one problem. Mr Cousins was disturbing the other patients with his laughter. He had, however, already arranged to move into an hotel room, which brought serenity and freedom from hospital routine. Dr Hitzig had been cautious about vitamin C, pointing out that claims for its efficacy in a wide range of diseases were controversial and that large doses could be harmful. Cousins decided to go ahead all the same, and began with an intravenous injection of 10 grammes. This too was followed by a drop in ESR. Cousins became convinced that the injections and laughter were both helping to defeat his illness. The dosage of vitamin C was increased. The laughter routine continued in full force. Cousin's fever receded, his pulse no longer raced, and sleep was becoming increasingly prolonged. After eight days he could move his thumbs without pain. Two weeks later his wife took him to the sunshine of Puerto Rico, and within a few days Norman Cousins was standing unaided in the surf. In less than a week he could not only walk but jog for a minute or two.

The infirmities did not disappear overnight, and it was some months before Cousins could get his arms up high enough to reach for a book on a high shelf. But he was back working full-time at the *Saturday Review*, and year by year since then his mobility has improved. Finally, in the year before he wrote his account, he became totally free of pain except in his knees. He was riding horses, playing tennis, and able to perform on the organ keyboard again.

What conclusions can we draw from such a story? A sceptic would dismiss the therapeutic value of laughter as a nonsense, scarcely worthy of consideration. Conventional medicine knows nothing of such tomfoolery. Intravenous doses of vitamin C of the size used here — reaching 25 grammes per day after three weeks — are known to be not only valueless but also positively hazardous. There is no evidence of a cause-and-effect relationship between exhaustion and the breakdown of collagen. And Mr Cousins's amateur speculation about the jet exhaust at Moscow airport can easily be written off as ill informed nonsense.

It would be more sensible, given this amazing account of the defeat of a condition for which mainstream medical science has no explanation, to pay attention to what the patient has to say. His two conclusions are sane and convincing. First, he believes that the will to live is not a theoretical abstraction but a physiological reality with therapeutic potential. He refused to accept the expert prognosis, so was not trapped in the cycle of fear, depression and panic that often accompanies supposedly incurable illness. While fully aware of the seriousness of his state — being unable to move his body was proof enough of that — he believed, deep down, that he had a good chance. So Cousins insists, from unique personal experience, on the ability of the patient, properly motivated, to participate actively in reversing disease or disability. Modern, rational medicine, founded securely on specific aetiology, does not rate such personal resources as important. It may even inhibit their expression.

The other conclusion from the central character in this rare story centres on his gratitude to a doctor who felt that *his* most useful response was to go along with his patient's ideas, encouraging to the full his will to live and his efforts to mobilise his own inner strength. 'Dr Hitzig was willing to set aside the large and often hazardous armamentarium of powerful drugs available to the modern physician when he became convinced that his patient had something better to offer,' Cousins writes. 'He was also wise enough to know that the art of healing is still a frontier profession . . . I would say that the principal contribution made by my doctor to the taming, and possibly the conquest, of my illness was that he encouraged me to believe I was a respected partner with him in the total undertaking.'

The most telling reflection on orthodox medicine's stance on such occasions is in the comments from several doctors who opined that Norman Cousins was probably the beneficiary of a mammoth venture in the self-administration of placebos. Cousins is happy to concede that this might well be true. Perhaps his belief in the value of vitamin C, not the vitamin itself, contributed to his getting well. But that would not account for his recovery, any more than the term 'spontaneous remission' explains the disappearance of cancer. We are still left with the challenge of healing that is beyond the explanatory scope of mechanistic medicine.

The Ringberg-Clinic

The relationship between healing, medical care, and scientific therapy is illustrated by the row which broke out in Britain in 1970-1 over the work of the Ringberg-Clinic run by Dr Josef Issels in Bavaria. Following a BBC television film which publicised (but did not adjudicate upon) the allegedly high cancer cure rates being achieved at the clinic, there was concern that Dr Issels might have devised methods of treatment that could be applied elsewhere. Experts were unconvinced that there was any value in his techniques, which included sera, dental extractions, and other measures designed to boost his patients' physical and psychological resources to thwart the disease. But, as a result of public clamour, a team of six senior British doctors visited the clinic to assess its methods and in due course published a report.

In the event, the committee found no conclusive evidence of above-average success rates. In fact Issels did not keep his patients' records in a style which would have allowed statistically valid comparisons to be made with conventional treatment elsewhere. From a scientific standpoint, therefore, the mission was a failure. Dr Issels apparently did not have a new magic bullet. But the committee had more to say than that. One of its conclusions was that 'the psychological approach to seriously ill patients is good; they are full of gratitude. Something active is being done for them, hope and encouragement are well given and they participate themselves in the effort made.' The doctor-patient relationship, the committee concluded, was 'very remarkable. Dr Issels and his patients become partners in a venture to try to save the patient's life.' Some patients lost their pain with reassurance alone, without drugs. They were often 'mentally and morally renewed'.

From the standpoint of materialist medicine, such achievements are insignificant. All that matters about malignant disease is whether or not a specific antidote is available. For most cancer patients — and their relatives — there is much more to it than that. Even without any quantifiable improvement in their condition, the understanding and humanity with which they are treated are of paramount importance.

Creative malady

The factor so often missing in scientific medicine is an appreciation of the interplay between a person and his or her illness — an error untraceable in the Hippocratic traditions which made no such distinction. An illustration of this is the way patients respond to and even make use of their afflictions. After a lifetime spent studying hypertension and other orthodox topics, Sir George Pickering has made an intriguing scrutiny of ill health in the famous and has come up with much evidence about hidden uses of debility. Charles Darwin, for example, was bothered by poor health all his life and among the speculations put forward to account for this is the idea that he suffered from Chagas's disease, a trypanosome infection acquired in March 1835 when he was bitten by the great black bug of the Pampas while crossing the Cordillera in Chile. In his book *Creative Malady* Pickering shows that this was most unlikely. A more plausible explanation is that Darwin turned into a solitary invalid simply to get on with his work. So too with Florence Nightingale, whose great achievement in stirring officialdom to the plight of the British soldier, after her return from the Crimea in 1856, was possible only because she became a bedridden recluse unable to see visitors and protected even from visits by her tiresome mother and sister.

Marcel Proust's story is more complex. He was wounded for life, apparently, when one day as a small boy his mother failed to kiss him goodnight as usual. He was always troubled by asthma, but immediately after his mother's death when he was thirty-four Proust became seriously ill and increasingly neurotic. Only later, after a friend stabbed his own mother to death, did he set out to prove that 'all men kill their mothers'. Though he and his mother had had an apparently deep, loving relationship, 'their love had been a mockery, because he had never forgiven that fatal omission of a goodnight kiss'.

With Mary Baker Eddy, Pickering writes, her 'agony of mind, expressed in her disabling illness, vanished when she began to sense what was to be her great contribution to thought and religion, namely the effect of mind on health . . . Christian science was a form of mental catharsis which was part of the cure of her illness.' From these and other case histories, he concludes that 'a psychoneurosis represents passion thwarted, a great creative work, passion fulfilled.' What is surprising is that such a verdict comes from a man who, throughout a long and distinguished career in mainstream medical science, has scarcely been a great enthusiast for the idea of psychosomatic disease.

Matter over mind

Just as difficult to fathom as psychological factors that may precipitate physical disease — or relieve it — is our vague awareness that infection is often accompanied or followed by depression. The fact that virus meningoencephalitis predisposes the victim to psychoses is scarcely surprising, because this is an affliction of brain tissue. But any virus infection — particularly influenza — may be succeeded for weeks or months by an incapacitating depression or anxiety even though the illness itself is mild and there is no evidence that the microbe has invaded the nervous system. Such is the impression gained by doctors experienced in treating virus infections and their repercussions. But proof is remarkably difficult to obtain. One recent study, by Drs M. Cadie, F. J. Nye and P. Storey, illustrates the problems. The investigators tried to find out, by both questionnaires and subjective interviews, how prevalent were depression and anxiety after glandular fever. They reached the perplexing conclusion that women were affected but men were not. Once again, our tools for inquiring into a not uncommon phenomenon are found wanting.

Our impotence to either understand or deal with such conditions is exemplified by an editorial in the *British Medical Journal* as recently as August 1976, which begins with a quotation from *The Nine Taylors* by Dorothy L. Sayers: 'Tell him to keep his spirits up. Such a nasty depressing complaint'. The treatment for influenzal depression suggested in this exhortation by the rector of Fenchurch St Pauls often proves to be lamentably inadequate, as the *British Medical Journal* concedes: 'The medium to long term prognosis may be good, but at the time depression may be profound and the suicidal risk real.' And the answer? 'Explanation and assurance of an eventually complete recovery are important and sometimes sufficient treatment, but a period of treatment with tricyclic antidepressants may be necessary.'

Subject and object

The problems we have considered so far underline the need for doctors to be very much more aware of psychological factors during their work. There are many other illustrative examples. Thus one research project has shown that 48.7 per cent of patients fail to take antibiotic tablets they have been prescribed.

Why, after feeling the need for a consultation, and having had the encounter sanctified by the handing over of a scientific cure, do half of us then neglect to consume what the expert ordered? Is the act of seeing a doctor more meaningful than ingestion of the remedy? Again, some psychologically disturbed patients deliberately and repeatedly mutilate themselves, often with great severity, yet experience not pain but relief and a decrease of tension. Why? And what lessons does this provide for the management of pain resulting from non-psychiatric illness? Between a sixth and a quarter of the adult population of Britain is plagued by sleep disorders; three and a half million people in England and Wales sleep with the aid of pills. Why? Is this pharmacological solution likely to be harmful?

These and many other questions, from bed wetting to patients' responses to hospital admission, from malingering to the spontaneous remission of a tumour, call for a greater appreciation of individual psychology. They are assuredly not problems that are likely to succumb to rational analysis built upon foundations of specific aetiology. Indeed, calculated suspension of rationality may be needed to throw light on riddles which have evaded, and will probably continue to evade, the rigorous searchlight of objectivity.

'The student of mind, for instance the practical psychiatrist at the mental hospital, must find the physiology of the brain still remote and vague for his desiderata on his subject,' wrote Sir Charles Sherrington in his classic *Man on his Nature* in 1940. He continues:

He may have hoped from it some knowledge which would serve to found the norm from which psycho-pathology could take its points of departure in this direction or in that. There is for instance the condition 'anxiety'. None is I suppose more far-reaching as a warper of the mind. But where does neurophysiology contribute anything to the knowledge of the norm from which anxiety causes departure and what has cerebral physiology to offer on the subject of 'anxiety'? The psychiatrist has perforce to go on his way seeking things more germane to what he needs.

Sherrington's purpose in his book was to explore the relationship between neurophysiology (study of the chemical and physical events in the brain) and consciousness. How does a thought, a memory, a feeling of anger or warmth or optimism, relate to changes in the cells in different regions of the brain? Sherrington did not solve the problem, and nearly four decades later we have made not one jot of progress towards an explanation. *Man on his Nature* remains the most elegant analysis of a puzzle, spanning the worlds of science and philosophy, which will probably never be solved. With the exception of a few diseases such as phenylketonuria, we are also no further forward in accounting mechanistically for much mental illness than when Sherrington highlighted the failure of his own scientific discipline to contribute to the description of anxiety. Where we have made a mistake, however, is in supposing there to be no benefit in the passage of ideas in the opposite direction. While physical medicine has relatively little to offer the psychiatrist and psychologist in grappling with the great mass of mental ill health, psychology used with intelligence and sensitivity may bring rich rewards in the understanding of physical illness.

It is scarcely surprising that this has not been realised, because most of those concerned with treating mental illness have themselves become polarised into separate cells of the medical enterprise. On the one hand there are the exponents of physical treatments. Following the pioneering work of Dr William Sargant in Britain, they rely almost entirely on drug therapy and such procedures as ECT. Leucotomy is the ultimate physical remedy. On the other hand there are the various schools of psychoanalysis and psychotherapy. They include the followers of Freud, Adler and Jung and, in the present day, figures such as R. D. Laing with his existential approach and Thomas Szasz who teaches that the mad are saner than the sane. They eschew drugs and physical techniques as violently as Dr Sargant and his disciples repudiate psychotherapy.

Three points are particularly significant about this conflict for our wider theme of specialisation and specific aetiology. First, the majority of drugs employed by the pharmacological enthusiasts, whatever their effects, non-effects, or side-effects, only masquerade as specific therapy. No one understands how the tranquillisers, prescribed in such gargantuan quantities, actually work. More is known about the antidepressant drugs, but only a little. There is no precise cause-and-effect relationship between their action on the nervous system and the relief of depression. Even the once popular categorisation of reactive (the consequence of external events) and endogenous (originating within the body) depression is no longer trusted. Most practitioners and most pharmaceutical advertisements imply otherwise, but therapy is, for the most part, empirical and non-specific.

Second, practitioners on both sides can invariably brandish evidence of patients they have helped who have previously, and disastrously, been attended by someone of the opposite persuasion. Third—and this is a comment on such 'casualty lists'—some of the most effective exponents of psychiatry are eclectic in their approach. They can see that neither side has a monopoly of insight or of therapeutic know-how. The mind is, in Sherrington's words, 'something with such manifold variety, such fleeting changes, such heights and depths of mood, such countless nuances, such sweeps of passion, such vistas of imagination' that it is unsurprising to find different patients responding differently to different therapies. With only a few exceptions, like phenylketonuria and general paralysis of the insane (syphilitic invasion of the nervous system), mental illness is not a subject of exact science.

The principle of complementarity

Schizophrenia provides one striking example of the two

radically different approaches to mental illness. R. D. Laing
describes schizophrenia in this way:

> The individual's being is cleft in two, producing a dis-
> embodied self and a body that is a thing that the self looks
> at, regarding it at times as though it were just another thing
> in the world. The total body and also many 'mental' pro-
> cesses are severed from the self, which may continue to
> operate in a very restricted enclave (fantasysing and observ-
> ing), or it may appear to cease to function altogether (i.e.
> be dead, murdered, stolen) . . . To the schizophrenic, liking
> someone equals *being like* that person: being like a person is
> equated with being the same as that person, hence with
> losing identity.

Now listen to Dr J. R. Smythies, a psychiatrist from the
University of Alabama Medical Center, reviewing recent
chemical hypotheses to account for the disease. One proposal
is the 'transmethylation hypothesis', according to which
'schizophrenia might be related to an aberration of trans-
mitter metabolism with the production in the body of compounds like mescalin. Other candidates for the possible
endogenous psychotoxin are similarly methylated derivates of
5-hydroxytryptamine such as dimethyltryptamine and 5-
methoxy-N,N-dimethyltryptamine'. An alternative notion is
that 'some cases of schizophrenia may be associated with an
imbalance between the brain dopamine systems (overactive)
and 5-hydroxytryptamine systems (underactive)'. After describing three other explanations for the origin of schizophrenia,
Smythies concludes that various forms of schizophrenia may
turn out to have distinct abnormal biochemistries.

There is no *necessary* conflict between Laing's description of
the disease and the attempt by Smythies to identify its
metabolic locus. In practice, however, practitioners of the two
persuasions do approach the problem very differently. Laing
tries to understand and to treat schizophrenia by psychoanalysis, by talking at length to his patients in the Hippocratic

manner, by seeking to identify closely with their inner world, and by searching for clues in their social behaviour and their intercourse with their families. The biochemists employ gas chromatography and mass spectrometry to scavenge body fluids for atypical metabolites — for 'psychotoxins' bearing the same specific relationship to the disease that the diphtheria toxin has to diphtheria. And while the Laing school can point to achievements in using 'therapeutic communities' to help liberate schizophrenics from their troubled state, biochemistry has yielded some successes too. Smythies describes one such case. She was a sixteen-year old girl diagnosed as schizophrenic who had a specific defect in a specific enzyme — $5^1,10^1$ methylenetetrahydrofolate reductase. She was cured by doses of folic acid, presumably because this corrected an underlying metabolic disorder. Moreover, many paranoid schizophrenics who formerly had to be kept in hospital for long periods for their own and society's protection have been returned to the community in relative contentment by courtesy of a group of drugs called the phenothiazines. But such progress scarcely vindicates the idea of discrete causation. The action of these drugs is not clear or precise. They are used as empirically and with as little knowledge as the tranquillisers are given for less traumatic forms of mental illness, unhappiness and fretfulness.

As we saw in Chapter 3, specific aetiology matched beautifully the determinism which dominated nineteenth-century science. The universe, it then seemed, was governed by cause and effect, by reactions opposed by equal and opposite reactions, by quantitative exactitude in the way matter and forces behaved. But with the arrival of Albert Einstein's relativity, Werner Heisenberg's uncertainty, and a handful of other historic discoveries in the first decades of the twentieth century, we learned that the universe is much more complex, its processes more elusive, than we had supposed. Beneath order is randomness, and our efforts to investigate the underlying phenomena are limited by inevitable, inbuilt deficiencies in our observational techniques. One concept that came out of this revolution in physics was that of complementarity. It was originally conceived as necessary to account for conflicting evidence about the electron, one of the constituents of the atom. Some experiments showed conclusively that the electron was a particle. Others proved beyond doubt that electrons manifested themselves as waves. Our experience of everyday events gives us no conceptual tools for grasping the fact that something can behave as both a particle and a wave. But that conclusion is unavoidable, so the Danish physicist Niels Bohr introduced the idea of complementarity to accommodate the paradox. The complementarity principle says that elementary matter consists of neither waves nor particles; but that when we examine matter we cannot avoid distorting it into looking like one or the other. Thus out of the 'hardest' science, physics, comes confirmation that there is a subjective element in all of our observations of nature. What we see depends upon our point of view.

Perhaps we should borrow the principle of complementarity to account for a disease like schizophrenia. Perhaps the psychodynamic and biochemical analyses are not opposed but complementary, each being valid within the observer's own terms. Such an approach would still leave the antagonists on each side arguing, but would free us of the mind-body dualism which, partnered by specific aetiology, has been so conspicuously unhelpful in illuminating the foundations of mental illness.

Mind-body dualism, though it goes back at least to Egyptian civilisation, was enunciated most clearly in Western culture by René Descartes in the seventeenth century. He taught that man consisted of two distinct parts: mind and body. The body was a physical object, like any other object in the world. The mind was the ego, with its thoughts and feelings. Extension in space was the criterion that distinguished the two; physical objects—brains included—were extended in space, mental objects were not. The riddle of how mind and brain interact, the problem that preoccupied Sir Charles Sherrington, has never been solved. Cartesian dualism has continued, however, to influence medicine and science—in part through the attempts that have been made to escape from an analysis uneasily suspected of being inadequate. Sir John Eccles, for example, has sought to do so by speaking of the brain harbouring 'a detector that has a sensitivity of a different kind from that of any physical instrument'. Others have contrived equally ingenious but unconvincing explanations for a link between two domains which, despite such exertions, are still conceived as distinct and separate. Competing with these ideas has been the rival theory of 'psychophysical monism', according to which mind simply does not exist. Thoughts and feelings are no more than electrochemical events in brain cells.

It is difficult to adjudicate over the degree of damage done by dualism and monism in fostering a simplistic medical approach to mind and body. What is clear is that neither rings true or provides a helpful framework for contemplating mental illness, whether serious or trivial, or 'psychosomatic' disease. Complementarity, which envisages consciousness and matter as different aspects of the same thing, seems a more satisfying basis. It has been well expressed by Professor Charles Coulson: 'Mind and matter are different ways of looking at the same set of phenomena, or experiences (i.e. man). Mind is not a sort of "ghost in the machine" called matter. Man is matter, or mind, according to the situation you are describing, and the pattern within which you give it meaning.'

Crime, chromosomes and causality

Let us now turn to two problems that have arisen out of a belief in strict causality in mental abnormality: the assessment of criminal responsibility and the adjustment of behavioural 'defects' by brain surgery. The first was precipitated by discoveries about the chromosomes that determine sex. Normal females have two X chromosomes in their cells, whereas males have one X and one Y chromosome. There are also several odd XY mixtures which produce conditions intermediate between femininity and masculinity. One abnormality has attracted particularly close scrutiny—the combination of one X with two Y chromosomes, first reported from the USA in 1961. Intense interest in XYY males was not aroused until 1965, however, when a study on inmates in the Scottish State Hospital, Carstairs—a maximum security hospital containing men convicted of violent crimes—revealed that about 3 per cent had XYY chromosomes. The frequency in the general population was thought to be about 0.1 per cent. Further, about one in four patients in the hospital who were six feet or more in height had two Y chromosomes. In the following year, examination of 50 men measuring six feet or over at two similar institutions showed that no less than 12 were XYY males. The implication that XYY individuals were thirty times more common in maximum security hospitals led to a considerable furore because of the supposed link between chromosomes and criminality. The extra Y chromosome seemed to threaten concepts of criminal liability and justice. If some people were driven to crime by specific chromosomes, rather than by conscious choice, or even environmental handicap, they must be correspondingly less culpable.

Further studies of the men in the Scottish State Hospital appeared to confirm these thoughts. All were severe psychopaths. And compared with other psychopaths from the same hospital, matched for age, height and IQ, but with normal chromosomes, the XYY men had tended to commit more crimes against property than against persons and had been convicted first at an earlier age (13 as opposed to 18 years). Comparison of family backgrounds showed an even more striking contrast. The XYY males came from families without any evidence of crime, and from all social classes. They were often the 'black sheep' of their otherwise law-abiding families. The men with whom they were compared tended to have criminal backgrounds. So the men's genes, rather than their environment, looked to be of paramount importance.

Subsequent analyses have modified these initial findings— findings upon which it was claimed that XYY children should be identified and treated as potential criminals. Further surveys have suggested that XYY males are almost as common in the population at large as in mental institutions and prisons. Others have confirmed the original discovery of a statistically significant difference between the two groups. A more fundamental objection to the earlier, almost Calvinistic claims is that the alleged effect of the XYY chromosome complement — antisocial behaviour — undoubtedly occurs in all communities. It is the laws and public standards in different societies, and the vigilance of police forces, that determine the likelihood of such people being incarcerated in prison or hospital. Also, the first men to be examined were selected because of 'behavioural disturbances', and it is inevitable that the original researchers were dealing with people in whom any effect of a chromosome abnormality was likely to be most severe. In due course, XYY individuals came to light who had formed perfectly adequate, 'normal' social relationships and had certainly not turned to crime. A prudent assessment of the evidence to date implies that a relationship does exist between XYY chromosomes and criminality but that — like most genetically determined factors — its expression is heavily influenced by environment.

There remain those who wish to pursue the matter further. The US Center for the Study of Crime and Delinquency has funded an investigation, at Harvard Medical School, designed to discern with greater clarity what influence XYY chromosomes have on behaviour. Part of their plan was to identify children with the abnormal chromosomes and then monitor their conduct as they grew up. Parents were consulted. Some were told that their child had a potentially significant genetic abnormality. Some were informed specifically of the XYY defect and its possible implications.

The project encountered strong opposition from Dr Jon Beckwith and other scientists at Harvard, who criticised the research on its basic premise — 'that we can and should attempt to distinguish between the behaviour of groups of people on the basis of genetics'. More specifically, they point out the difficulty of determining whether an XYY child's behavioural problems are caused by his chromosomes or by the impact on the child-parent relationship of the information given to parents that their son has such an abnormality. Similar difficulties attend the withholding of information. By adhering to strictly scientific methods of experimentation, and observing the development of an XYY child without informing its parents, researchers might easily deny the child psychiatric or other assistance that could be helpful in coping with his problems. There appears to be no way around the central dilemma. Should such research proceed on the basis of parental knowledge and co-operation—with the likelihood that any results will be rendered uninterpretable because of information given to parents? Or should it be done in secrecy, possibly yielding meaningful conclusions, but with the risk of denying psychiatric aid to children in need? There seems to be no answer to the dilemma that is consistent with both scientific rigour and social compassion.

Psychosurgery and behaviour

Leucotomy, which began with the work of Egas Moniz (see p. 61), is the procedure of severing the tracts linking the prefrontal lobes with the rest of the brain, or the removal of more extensive parts of the frontal cortex. Its aim is thoroughly materialistic; to eradicate or block transmission of those mental messages which distress the patient or make him or her behave improperly. The earliest results were in turning deteriorated schizophrenics and violent patients into passive vegetables. The technique spread from Portugal to the USA and Britain during the 1940s and 1950s. In England and Wales in 1949, 1,200 patients were leucotomised. One study suggested that 46 per cent of those suffering from schizophrenia 'improved' after the operation, while 25 per cent were unchanged, and 4 per cent died. But a further investigation, which was more carefully controlled and in which the patients were followed up for several years, showed that the outcome did not differ significantly from that in non-leucotomised patients. Worse, the loss of a substantial area of brain seemed to produce a variety of deleterious results, including intellectual and emotional retardation, blunted creativity, selfishness and greed. For these reasons, the procedure fell into disrepute — but not before surgeons had experimented with the destruction of virtually every part of the brain that could be obliterated without killing the patient. By the time 'psychosurgery' went out of favour in the mid-1950s, an estimated 100,000 operations had been performed throughout the world.

In the late 1960s, leucotomy came back into favour, particularly in the USA. This time it was employed not to treat schizophrenics, but to deal with all manner of quasi-medical conditions — 'hyperactivity' in children, drug addiction, depression — and a wide variety of candidates — 'frigid' and 'promiscuous' women, aggressive prisoners, homosexuals. All were considered suitable for specific brain surgery. The practitioners responsible were surgeons who believed that, using more accurate and selective techniques, they could destroy discrete brain functions with far greater precision than was possible a decade earlier. Often, conventional surgery is unnecessary. Tissue can be inactivated by coagulating it electrically, by implanting radioactive 'seeds', or by freezing.

The medicalisation of social and psychological problems by chemotherapy is a retrograde step. How much more so when the technique is irreversible surgery? Such developments precipitated a great outcry in the United States in the early 1970s, led by a Harvard psychiatrist Dr Peter Breggin. There is some evidence that since then surgeons specialising in leucotomy have become more judicious in their criteria for selecting patients. But the temptations remain.

Does psychosurgery actually work as a means of coping with overt mental illness? A recent review of evidence which suggests the need for considerable caution is to be found in the Australian publication *The Magic Bullet*. Dr Jules Older points out that surgeons in this field tend to overstate their achievements. One Japanese team, for example, has claimed an improvement rate of nearly 70 per cent. But this figure includes young children, many of whom are likely to improve without treatment of any kind over the course of time. When those under twelve are excluded, the rate falls to 31 per cent. A leading Indian surgeon has published results in which he included among the 'improved' category patients who were 'manageable when given drugs though not leading a useful life'. Without this group, his apparent success rate fell from over 75 per cent to under 40 per cent. One American doctor listed a patient in his 'good result' group despite intellectual deterioration. And the mother of a patient described by a prominent American team as a qualified success sued the doctors for two million dollars, charging them with turning her son into a vegetable.

One difficulty in interpreting results from physical treatments for mental illness is that nearly every new technique seems to work, at least temporarily. Many such therapies have been tried, discarded, rediscovered, and discarded again over the last forty years. They include insulin shock therapy, vitamins, electrosleep, inhalation of nitrogen, and the use of LSD and other hallucinogens. Older writes:

> The effects of enthusiasm, the desire for good results, and the expectation of change have clouded the results of many an experiment, even those involving rats. When the subjects are suffering humans who are desperate for relief, the need for carefully designed research is even greater. Yet many studies of psychosurgery's effects have been marked by lack of controls, inadequate 'blindness' of the judges and shoddy criteria of success.

The outstanding argument in favour of caution is that long-term studies are essential before success can be claimed with assurance. One of the leading proponents of psychosurgery, Dr William Sweet, has said: 'It is clear that not only adverse but also favourable results may disappear and long follow-up periods are essential before final opinions are given.' Dr Older cites research on the effects of cingulotomy, one of the newer techniques now held to be most promising, showing that despite immediate improvement in most cases, the symptoms of half the patients return in the course of time: 'Although there have been some attempts at long-term follow-up studies, there is not yet clear evidence as to whether success of the new wave of psychosurgery will hold up over time.'

Who is supposed to benefit from psychosurgery? Are specific regions of brain tissue destroyed to help the patient, or to make life easier for his family or his prison officers? Among the indications that have been used as a basis for such operations on children are 'aggressive behaviour' and 'wandering tendencies'. One American funding proposal reported by Older, for the setting up of a prison unit incorporating both psychosurgery and aversion conditioning experiments, describes these procedures not as therapies but as means of controlling 'serious management problem inmates'. The spectre of psychosurgery in conformity with state norms may not be as remote as many people imagine. We do, after all, live in times that have seen the label 'schizophrenia' used to justify incarceration and to still political dissent in the Soviet Union.

Such thoughts are undoubtedly far from the minds of most surgeons who have been experimenting with leucotomy. It is, nevertheless, disquieting to find one British enthusiast, Dr R. F. Tredgold, using the following sentences to complete a review of results he and his colleagues have achieved:

> It should be pointed out that relatively few patients in our series had had full-scale psychotherapy. Whether this would have been equally or more successful than operation is another unanswered question. But what can be said is that it is most unlikely that psychotherapy of the skill and intensity required will be available for many such cases in mental hospitals in the foreseeable future.

Dr Tredgold is a man of the highest professional integrity, but it is a disturbing reflection of the current situation that, whatever the value or demerits of leucotomy, facilities for patients to be dealt with by the alternative psychotherapeutic approach are inadequate.

The healing tradition

Although specific aetiology has yielded only a vanishingly small number of insights in understanding or treating mental illness, the concept has had a considerable influence on this sector of medicine. Whether in supporting the notion that misbehaviour can be corrected by obliterating discrete regions of the brain, or in the less sinister administration of chemical tranquillisers to cope with personal problems, the notion of specificity continues to be a powerful motif. But perhaps its most damning effect has often been to divert attention away from the personal factors that seem of such grossly underestimated significance in health and disease. Not only in psychosomatic illness, but also in those diseases which orthodox medicine believes it has exhaustively described and delineated, individual psychology can be a potent force. Whether that force is mobilised in the patient, whether it is recognised by the doctor, whether it atrophies amidst the clinical sophistication of scientific medicine, are questions that point up the contrast between precision therapy and the Hippocratic tradition of healing.

6
Health, class and country

So far, we have inspected the paradoxical inadequacies of scientific medicine's central tenet in accounting for some of the ills that plague mind and body. In the next three chapters, we turn to three more radical defects of specific aetiology. These are positive demerits rather than mere failures. First, by focusing attention on mechanical and metabolic malfunctioning in individuals, the great but flawed theory has induced us to ignore the wider insights that can be gleaned by seeing health and ill health from the perspective of the community. Second, it has encouraged a narrow preoccupation with the treatment of disease rather than the maintenance of health. Third, it has fathered a style of Western medical practice whose deficiencies and distortions become vividly apparent when it is exported to the Third World. These shortcomings are interconnected. Together, they amount to a weighty indictment of the conceptual and practical tool with which over the past century doctors and scientists have carried through a medical revolution. Specific aetiology, I shall argue in the final chapter, is an idea that has had its day.

Writing in Bukhara over nine hundred years ago, Al Asuli divided his pharmacopoeia into two parts. They were headed 'Diseases of the Rich' and 'Diseases of the Poor'. He recognised, albeit at a time when few ailments were defined properly and when even fewer could be cured, that there were social distinctions in the pattern of ill health. The notion did not prosper, however, and it was eclipsed totally a century ago by the infinitely more powerful interpretation afforded by the germ theory. Only very recently have we begun to hear serious talk of 'diseases of affluence', and departments of 'social medicine' are few and far between. But at its twenty-ninth World Health Assembly, meeting in Geneva in May 1976, the World Health Organisation affirmed that psychosocial factors should be taken into account in health programmes and the delivery of health care. The Belgian Minister of Health, Mr J. de Saeger, said this was 'a new dimension or, if you like, a new inspiration, giving new life to all our activities'.

Mapping cardiovascular disease

The widest canvas for viewing ill health in relation to community comprises the comparatively young discipline of medical geography. Following the frustrating failure of laboratory studies to pinpoint the cellular origins of conditions such as cancer and coronary heart disease, investigators have begun to pore over profiles of these maladies in different countries and different societies. Central to medical geography is the painstaking comparison of morbidity statistics and the search for clues in regional climatic, social, environmental and other factors. Where the narrow focus has revealed little, this broader analysis may succeed. The returns so far have been small, but there are high hopes that the novel technique will win rich rewards.

Disease of the heart and blood vessels poses one tantalising problem. Although the statistical evidence is poor, we know that total mortality from cardiovascular conditions is very small in developing countries. This is true even when we allow for the younger age structure of the populations. Yet, as we have seen, this same affliction is now the commonest cause of death in Western societies. Are white people peculiarly disposed to heart disease? Some evidence supports the idea, but against it is the fact that Negroes in America are much more prone to heart trouble than people in most of Africa and India. The real explanation seems to lie in diet and lifestyle (see p. 80).

In 1974 the World Health Organisation drew up for the first time a 'heart map' of Europe. It shows that the northern and north-western countries have the highest frequencies of heart attacks, while the southern areas escape most lightly. The rate in Helsinki and Tampere, Finland, is five times greater than in Sofia, Bulgaria, with a gradual reduction traceable on the map from north to south. The medium incidence zone includes Holland, the Federal Republic of Germany, Czechoslovakia, Poland and Hungary. The map was based on the records of every heart attack in 1971-2, and as all the regions studied have excellent medical services the figures are highly dependable.

Thus a geographical perusal of morbidity statistics can throw up information which would never come to light in the laboratory. The next, obvious, question concerns the variations — in weather, perhaps, or geology, or social behaviour — which account for the crude divergences. One suspect factor is drinking water. In 1957, Dr J. Kobayashi reported that he had found a close association between deaths from cardiovascular disease in Japan and the acidity of the river water used for drinking. People who consumed water that was more alkaline had a correspondingly smaller risk of dying from this cause. Dr H. A. Schroeder followed up the clue in the United States by comparing mortality figures with information about the hardness of the water in different areas. (Generally speaking, the more acidic the water, the softer it is.) The results confirmed what Dr Kobayashi had discovered in Japan: the softer the water, the higher the death rate from cardiovascular disease. Dr Schroeder noticed other associations, between, for example, water hardness and cirrhosis of the liver, but the outstanding finding was the relationship of soft water to heart disease.

Dr M. D. Crawford has confirmed a very similar picture in

Britain. It is highlighted in Glasgow and the other Scottish cities; all have extremely soft water together with high cardiovascular death rates. Of other causes of death, there was also a significant correlation between bronchitis and water softness. This is not surprising, as many bronchitics die of cardiac complications, and the two labels are sometimes confused or interchanged on death certificates. One intriguing sidelight to emerge from Dr Crawford's study is an explanation of the previously perplexing observation that coronary heart disease — a condition associated with affluence — causes more deaths in Glasgow and north-country textile towns than anywhere else in the country. These centres are far from affluent — but they have extremely soft water. Overall, Dr Crawford estimates that if the cardiovascular mortality rates seen in towns with very hard water applied throughout Britain, there would be about 4,000 fewer deaths each year among men in the 45-64 age group alone.

These results do not, of course, prove definitively that drinking soft water makes one more likely to develop heart disease. There are grounds for being cautious about such an interpretation. One research project in Oklahoma and another in Ireland revealed no association between coronary disease and the softness of drinking water. On the other hand again, both of these surveys were conducted with very small populations. A more recent investigation has confirmed the earlier relationship in different parts of Ontario, while a wider study in Ireland has shown some correlation in the same direction. From the overall pattern, it seems that the softness of drinking water is indeed significant in cardiovascular disease. It is one more 'risk factor' to be added to those we considered in Chapter 4.

Causes of cancer

Although cancer is a universal affliction its frequency in different organs and tissues varies dramatically throughout the world. In contrast to the stance of much laboratory science, founded on a unitary approach and a search for 'the cause', field and geographical studies suggest that we should consider every type of cancer separately. Thus malignant tumours of the liver and mouth are more common in southern Africa and India than in Europe or North America. The opposite is true for cancer of the large intestine.

Cancer of the lung and windpipe is widespread in the USA, USSR, and central and eastern Europe, and appears to be commoner in Britain than anywhere else in the world. The disease is almost unknown in east and west Africa, but recently it has become one of the most frequently diagnosed tumours among Africans in the towns of Zambia and South Africa. Many of these correlations — and the delayed but more rapid increase among women compared with men in Britain and the USA — suggest that cigarette smoking is to blame. But as we have seen (p. 82) the picture lacks clarity and certainty.

One of the most baffling puzzles is the distribution of stomach cancer, which is widespread throughout Soviet Asia but reaches its highest prevalence in Japan. The disease declines gradually westwards, falling to a much lower level in North America. Iceland is atypical, with a high incidence, while distribution is somewhat irregular in the southern hemisphere. Two clues might help to account for this pattern. First, the Japanese population of Hawaii has far less stomach cancer than that in Japan. This implies that environmental or dietary, rather than genetic, influences are of prime importance. Second, the prevalence of the disease has dropped in recent years in North America and Europe — against the trend for most other tumours. A suggested explanation is that carcinogenic materials are liberated when foodstuffs deteriorate — something which has been combated by refrigeration and improved techniques of food preservation.

A story of detection

The pattern of oesophageal cancer in different parts of Africa is another puzzling irregularity. Some years ago Dr A. G. Oettlé showed that even south of the Sahara the distribution of this tumour was extremely patchy. In his report he mentioned the possibility that lead or another metallic element was responsible, but he could not relate the disease to any known physical factor in the environment. Indeed, areas of high incidence varied widely in their geographical characteristics. Correlations with both smoking and alcoholism were suspected, but there was no conclusive evidence either way.

The first breakthrough came when Dr R. J. W. Burrell plotted the homes of the cancer victims on a large map of localities where the disease was relatively common. A marked 'clustering' was obvious immediately, with the patients' homes scattered around shebeens — stores of illicitly prepared spirits. Moreover, when the police identified and closed particular shebeens the pattern changed, to be replaced later by a localisation of cases around newly opened liquor stores. Many difficulties attended this and later work in pinpointing the cause of the clustering. One stemmed from the latent period of the cancer: the social customs responsible for a disease pattern are not necessarily those prevailing at the time when it is investigated. Another was the reluctance of cancer victims in some parts of Africa to seek treatment. The Bantu, for example, are often fatalistic when stricken by a condition they believe to be incurable, and they may elect deliberately to die at home without receiving medical attention. Such cases do not then appear in the hospital records scrutinised in statistical surveys.

Faced with these problems, Dr Neil McGlashan and a team from the University of Zambia initiated a survey in central Africa in 1965 designed to gather hard statistics about oesophageal cancer and its relationship to environmental and social factors. Even during the 8,000-mile journey, a clear correlation began to emerge between the tumour and consumption of the illicit liquor known as *kachasu* or Malawi gin. The team collected samples for testing later. At the end of the safari, a statistically valid correlation was amply confirmed, and the investigators sent their samples to the laboratory for chemical analysis.

Kachasu is distilled from a beverage of maize, maize cobs, and sugar. The crude equipment used for the job is usually knocked up from old metallic containers, with bicycle frames and discarded exhaust pipes as condensers. Analysis revealed wide variations in the composition of the spirits, but the better quality preparations contained up to 30 per cent of alcohol. Some samples had high levels of zinc (which was traced to the galvanised iron drums used as fermentation vessels) and copper (from tubing and to a larger extent contamination with copper-rich soil). The content of these metals could, therefore, account for the cancer—and there were suspicions that the use of metallic tubes and containers was related in time to the increase in oesophageal cancer over the previous twenty-five years. This hypothesis, however, did not last long. Visits to parts of Zambia where oesophageal cancer was rare showed that local alcoholic drinks were just as heavily contaminated with copper or zinc or both.

Then came some crucial news. Chemists at the British Food Manufacturing Industries' Research Association, Leatherhead, had detected minute amounts of a carcinogen, dimethyl-N-nitrosamine (DMN), in the earlier Zambian samples. Next, a survey further afield (including Ghana, Eire, Canada, and Yugoslavia) showed that wherever spirits were prepared by illegal distillation, necessitating secrecy and crude methods, the final product contained DMN. But where did it come from? The investigators returned to Kenya, where they had found the highest concentrations of DMN in any of their samples, and tested the separate ingredients used at each stage of manufacture. The result: DMN was absent from all the starting materials but appeared during fermentation. It probably originated from wild yeasts which, in dirty conditions, can easily contaminate a fermentation brew.

Another piece of the jigsaw emerged during a visit to the Mazandaran province of northern Iran to investigate the high incidence of oesophageal cancer there, particularly among women. In this devout Muslim area alcohol could not be responsible for the tumour. But the research team found DMN in grape vinegar (made by fermentation); pickles prepared using the vinegar; and anarteen, a mixture concocted from raisins, pomegranate seeds, and black peppercorns which is taken to relieve digestive discomfort during pregnancy.

I have chosen this example because it illustrates both the strengths and weaknesses of specific aetiology. The episode can be compared with John Snow's demonstration, almost exactly a century earlier, of the spread of cholera via the Broad Street pump. Yet it would not have reached a successful conclusion had the investigators not relinquished the straitjacket with which medical science enveloped itself following the dramatic triumphs of the germ theory. Snow was a natural historian of disease, an epidemiologist who adopted a social perspective. But many of his successors, dazzled by triumphs in applying simplistic concepts of disease, renounced that wider view. The link between DMN and oesophageal cancer came not just from science but from sociology too. Laboratory technology alone would never have solved the problem. It would not even have shown the problem to exist.

Cancer and lifestyle

So too with the striking correlation between comparative affluence and the incidence of bowel and breast cancer. Both of these tumours are far more common in the West than in developing countries. Specific aetiology was of no value to us in discerning this relationship, let alone in investigating it further. The two conditions appear to be encouraged greatly by the Western lifestyle, with diet as the chief suspect. In the case of bowel cancer, either a shortage in the diet of the fibrous indigestible residue we term roughage (see p. 158) or excess fat may be responsible. The dietary evidence is less certain for breast cancer, though the indications are there. Why, for example, should Japanese women, who seldom develop breast tumours, increase their chances of doing so when they move to the United States and adopt a new way of life?

Lifestyle seems particularly influential in those forms of cancer that are related to hormones produced by the endocrine system in the body. Breast tumours, which kill more women in the USA than any other variety, and prostate cancer, which follows only malignancies of the lung and bowel as a cause of death among men, are the two main examples. According to Dr John Berg, of the University of Iowa:

> The most plausible hypothesis, although based on extremely incomplete knowledge, is that some components of the Western high-protein, high-fat diet acting in early life make individuals prone to develop these cancers . . . In speculation one could go so far as to suggest that mankind generally evolved under conditions of prudent (i.e. low fat and protein) nutrition and that the present affluent diet from childhood onward may overstimulate the endocrine system, producing the same effect that one would obtain running a diesel engine on high-octane aeroplane fuel.

Uninteresting people?

Denis Burkitt, the surgeon who has publicised his belief in the significance of dietary fibre in reducing the likelihood of bowel cancer, and who also discovered the relationship between climatic factors in Africa and 'Burkitt's lymphoma', believes that areas of non-incidence are of key importance in cancer research. There may be more clues, he suggests, in regions that are comparatively free of cancers and such diseases as peptic ulcer and atherosclerosis than in those where these conditions are abundant. By that criterion, the most attractive place in the world for the cancer specialist should be the high plateaux of the Himalayas, north of Kashmir, in the Karakoram. The Hunza, the people who live there, appear to have no cancer whatever. A doctor working for the Indian Medical Service, Sir Robert McCarrison, discovered this incredible fact over half a century ago. At first, McCarrison found the Hunza very uninteresting because, apart from mending a few fractures, he had nothing to do when he was serving in the area. On reflection, though, he was greatly struck by the people's health. They suffered very little illness indeed and were entirely free of malignant disease. His observations, which met scepticism at first, have been confirmed by other investigators. The explanation, it seems, must be sought in the combination of a calm, stress-free life, a simple diet, which is rich in vitamins but otherwise frugal, and cleanliness and absence of industrial pollution.

The birth of geocancerology

In 1973, participants at an international symposium held in Brussels by the European Institute of Ecology and Cancer resolved to establish a discipline concerned with the geography of cancer, to stimulate the adoption of a wider approach to the disease. Termed 'geocancerology', the new branch of study embraces not only cartography and statistics, but also soil science, biosociology, ecology, town planning, and other specialities. Together, they may be able to throw light on conditions that so far have evaded adequate description as a result of their more individual attentions. Its aim is 'to study the influence of factors such as physical and social environment, mode of life and bio-anthropological make-up' on different forms of cancer, especially on their distribution and aetiology. Geography is the main tool, but one to be used alongside a synthesis of the other fields of study.

The English disease

An outstanding example of a condition that can be understood fully only in its social and environmental context is bronchitis. Strictly speaking, it is an infection. A particular bacterium, usually *Haemophilus influenzae*, damages the bronchial tubes, causing the characteristic cough and sputum production. And the medical journals are replete (especially during winter months) with advertisements for appropriate antibiotic preparations with which doctors can attack the invaders. Yet those same microorganisms—varieties we all carry in our respiratory tract from time to time without suffering in the least—can scarcely be described as the 'real' cause of bronchitis. For an accurate account of the disease we have to consider its geographical and social background.

Thus, although the microbes involved are universal, deaths from chronic bronchitis are thirty times more frequent in the United Kingdom than in the USA—and five or six times commoner than in most of Western Europe. Not surprisingly, this has been termed the English disease, and the blame has been attached to the country's damp, inhospitable climate. Even that is not the full story. Within Britain, bronchitis is largely a town disease, being rare in rural areas but widespread in industrial centres. It is also an affliction of the poor; mortality is highest among unskilled men and women and falls progressively to reach its lowest level among professional people.

Thus the memorable events in the story of bronchitis are not major epidemics triggered by the emergence of especially virulent strains of bacteria. They are episodes of horrendous air pollution, caused by the engines of industry, which kill people already suffering from the disease. One such episode occurred at Donora, south of Pittsburgh, in 1948, when there was a major fog and weather inversion. By the third day of the four-day incident, over 40 per cent of the people in Donora, a town in a river valley surrounded by hills, were affected by respiratory illness, with cough, sore throat, nasal discharge, smarting of the eyes, tears, nausea, headache, weakness, and occasional muscular aches and pains. Some reported vomiting and diarrhoea. Seventeen people died, most of them elderly or already troubled by heart and lung disease. Post mortems on five victims revealed bronchitis and abnormalities in the lung tissues indicating acute irritation. Such changes cannot tell us specifically which atmospheric pollutants were to blame, but it seems that there was a large amount of sulphur dioxide in the air at the time, together with airborne particles and other gases. As two medical ecologists, W. Harding le Riche and Jean Miller, have commented: 'To the pathologist the exact cause of this situation could not be demonstrated, while the epidemiologist was left with an impression and a great deal of suggestive evidence.'

Britain's most famous episode of atmospheric pollution was the London 'smog' of 5 - 9 December 1952, in which 4,000 people died. Many were bronchitics. One result of this historic smog was a public outcry, leading to the implementation of the Clean Air Act, which has eliminated the possibility of any such disasters in future. Another serious fog did hit London in 1962, but what are euphemistically termed the 'excess deaths' attributed to the pollution then numbered only 350 - 750. Although there was about the same amount of sulphur dioxide in the air on the two occasions, by 1962 the quantity of smoke in London had been reduced considerably.

But horrendous smogs do not cause bronchitis; they exacerbate it and kill chronic bronchitics whose respiratory tissues are already so ravaged by disease that they cannot withstand further massive assaults. What, then, is the *real* cause? Smoking is certainly an important contributor, and continual air pollution, overcrowded living conditions, and damp bedrooms have also been implicated. In 1972 Dr J. L. Girt published the results of a survey he carried out in one of Britain's northern industrial cities in an attempt to find out more. He studied over 700 women living in Leeds, asking them questions designed to discover their experience of chronic bronchitis (defined as 'the production of phlegm on most days for as much as three months in the year'). The sample was random, so that bronchitics were found independently of whether they themselves were aware of their condition or had sought treatment for it. The women also replied to queries about smoking habits and their past and present housing and employment.

Dr Girt chose Leeds, with its population of half a million, because the city contained most of the variations in housing and environment that might be significant for the prevalence of bronchitis. It grew to be a major industrial centre during the nineteenth century, developing clothing, engineering and chemical works. The river Aire, whose banks are occupied almost totally by industry, runs through Leeds from west to east. Industry extends from the city centre to a coalfield immediately south. So, while the southern half of the city is a mixture of industry and housing, the northern part is primarily residential. A high proportion of dwellings were built in the last century, and many back-to-back terrace houses remain, particularly in the industrial areas. In places they occur at densities of more than 6,800 to the square kilometre.

To study a representative range of environments, Dr Girt selected thirty localities, within which he approached random samples of householders. Only females were interviewed, partly for the convenience of contacting them during the daytime, but mainly because their occupational histories were expected to be simpler and shorter than those of the men. As bronchitis is primarily a disease of middle and later years, the survey had a lower age limit of fifteen.

The results were not altogether expected. Present-day levels of air pollution, and possibly those in the past as well, were not related to the women's risk of having chronic bronchitis. But cigarette smoking and the standard of housing, both past and present, were highly influential. 'We can lay the blame for the high incidence of bronchitis in Leeds among females on housing conditions and smoking,' Dr Girt concluded. 'It would appear that the disease is largely the result, excluding the effects of smoking, of small, inadequately constructed houses which, particularly in Victorian times, were produced in quantities to house the working man and his family.' Dr Girt's figures support this verdict, the disease being strongly associated with overcrowding and damp homes.

'Slum clearance' is thus endorsed as a means of combating chronic bronchitis. But that is not all. Also important are measures to minimise overcrowding and to secure high-quality building. 'We must hope that suburbanisation, rising living and housing standards, and the tendency to have smaller families will be continued for bronchitis to be beaten,' Dr Girt says. 'In Leeds, at least, and probably in most other cities as well, the solution lies in the hands of the local authorities.'

Clusters of illness

Specific aetiology has little to say about such effects of physical environment on disease. It is no more helpful in the realm of social environment. A study conducted by Dr L. E. Hinkle and his colleagues at the New York Hospital Cornell Medical Center has explored this area through the medical histories of several thousands of patients over a period of twenty years, which were taken and evaluated by a cultural anthropologist and a sociologist as well as by a psychiatrist and physician. A major conclusion was that our illnesses do not appear at random. They come in 'clusters', which may last for several years. Moreover—most significantly—they include diseases with, on a conventional understanding, widely differing aetiologies. In other words, there are periods in our lives when we are unusually prone not simply to influenza or low back pain or anxiety neurosis but to influenza *and* low back pain *and* anxiety neurosis. These clusters tend to occur at times when we have difficulty in coping with our environment as we see it. In each of three groups in the Cornell study (drawn from different social backgrounds) there were people who were usually healthy and others with a greater susceptibility to all illnesses. Each also included examples of clustered illnesses apparently triggered by an emotional stress such as bereavement.

Those who were most prone to ill health were those who had adapted least contentedly to their situation in life. It seems that all disease processes can be influenced by the way we adjust or fail to adjust to our social milieu. Yet mechanistic medicine has ignored these relationships almost totally.

Mental illness

Epidemiology, as the word implies, used to mean simply the charting and study of epidemics. Today, we speak of the epidemiology not only of infections but also of cancers and heart disease — and even of neuroses and psychoses. Surprisingly, this approach to mental illness has lagged behind its extension into other areas of non-infectious disease. Already, though, it has proved itself a legitimate tool. Thus the work of Lord Taylor and others in Britain has shown that neurotic symptoms (and also minor physical complaints) among families who have moved into 'new towns' are often more frequent than they were in the old, perhaps dilapidated, areas from which they came. An apparent improvement in physical environment does not necessarily promote health; the reverse may well apply.

Similarly, a study in Aberdeen by Sheila Bain, reported in 1973, showed that referral rates for all psychiatric disorders correlated with overcrowded conditions and, most strikingly, with a decrease in the number of persons in a household. She concluded that people were at greater risk in contracting mental illness in Aberdeen if they lived in areas of high population density but also where there were smaller numbers per household. There were also some intriguing contrasts with earlier surveys conducted in Chicago in the USA; in Mannheim, Germany; and in Nottingham in the UK. Each of these showed that the highest referral rates for all psychiatric disorders were in the inner core of these cities, centred on the slum and poorer industrial areas. This was not so in Aberdeen. The explanation, presumably, could be found in the different lifestyles of people in the Scottish city and those in the other three — and perhaps also in Aberdeen's much smaller industrial base. These are the sort of factors that only a geographical survey is able to probe.

But epidemiology deals not only with variations across space; it is concerned with time too. Why, for example, is the incidence of some psychosomatic conditions, and some of those suspected of having a psychosomatic origin, changing in the two sexes? It appears that peptic ulcer and hypertension, which in the nineteenth century were common in women, are now affecting an increasing proportion of men. Others, like diabetes, that were predominantly diseases of males in the last century, are now prevalent among females. Have these changes resulted from alterations in the roles of the sexes in Western society over the past fifty years?

Entire diseases, apparently specific maladies in their day, have disappeared. We no longer see epidemics of 'dancing mania', while the hysterical convulsion states of a century ago are now a rarity. Also little more than historical curiosities are involutional melancholia and agitated preoccupation with sinfulness. Hysterical conversion symptoms were common among soldiers in the First World War, but these were replaced by anxiety neurosis during the Second World War. Even some of the symptoms of schizophrenia, such as catatonic posturing, details of which were described clearly in medical textbooks a few decades back, are now almost unheard of. All of these developments are thought to stem not from any innate evolution in human behaviour but from alterations in the social environment.

Health and social class

Let us now shift our perspective somewhat, and see what we can learn about the pattern of disease in different social classes. An analysis of this sort is, of course, fraught with difficulties — not least that of defining social classes (and even, in these egalitarian days, conceding that they are meaningful). Suffice to say that the data do exist, and that statisticians and pollsters continue to divide people into five groups, ranging from senior professional and managerial families (social class I) to unskilled manual workers and their families (social class V). Perhaps the most disquieting evidence that such divisions are real is to be seen when medical data are marshalled accordingly. In Britain, almost all of the major causes of death, including coronary heart disease, lung cancer, cervical cancer, pneumonia and bronchitis, are commoner among people in social class V than in social class I. The number of deaths per year from these causes is 50 per cent higher in social classes IV and V combined (the bottom quarter of the population) than in social classes I and II combined (the top quarter). And the gap is widening both relatively and absolutely. It is now two or three times larger than during the early 1930s.

Richard Wilkinson, working in the Department of Community Health at Nottingham University, tried recently to identify the origin of these distinctions, by examining mortality figures for twenty different diseases and matching them with factors such as housing, incomes and jobs. His conclusion, based on a comprehensive computer analysis, was that housing conditions and occupational fatalities now make little difference to annual death rates. What he did find was a strong association of mortality rates and income. This seemed to be due almost entirely to a relationship with diet.

Such a conclusion may be scarcely surprising in view of the sort of information about British eating habits compiled in the National Food Survey. This shows that poor people eat 56 per cent less fruit per head than the rich, 19 per cent less fresh green vegetables, 21 per cent less milk, and 31 per cent less carcass meat. (The rich here are defined as those earning £5,000 a year or more in 1974, while the poor were earning £1,200 or less, and the figures are 11-year averages, from 1964-74.) The only apparent way in which the diet of the low wage earners is superior is in its slightly lower fat content. Otherwise — whatever dietary theory one favours — their food appears highly unbalanced, with huge calorie compensations in bread, sugar, and potatoes.

Wilkinson singles out six aspects of these nutritional distinctions which could account for the higher death rates among the poor. First, obesity is far commoner among the less well off. And obesity increases one's susceptibility to a very wide range of conditions as well as those, such as coronary heart disease, that are strikingly more prevalent in the overweight. Not an excess of calories, but too many calories from the wrong foods, seems to be the explanation. Second, poor people eat less fibre (indigestible vegetable matter) than do rich people — and fibre is now being recognised as important in protecting us against several diseases (see p. 158). Third, the poor receive less vitamins than the rich, which probably makes them more prone to infections. Fourth, their high sugar consumption may contribute to a greater risk of heart disease, atherosclerosis and diabetes. Fifth, the trace elements found in fruit, vegetables, milk and meat are thought to be important to health — and these foods too are more plentiful in the diets of the better off. Finally, there is some evidence that vitamins and other constituents that are commoner in upper-class diets may retard the development of atherosclerosis.

The evidence implicating these factors in health and disease is far from clear-cut, as Wilkinson concedes. But between them they offer a promising explanation for his overall findings. Wartime experiences confirm the general picture. In the First World War, the British people learned the hard way about the danger to health posed by an inadequate diet. These lessons were applied during the Second World War, when the government introduced rationing but arranged by scrupulous calculation that everyone received enough of certain essential nutrients. So although sugar and fat consumption fell, particularly during the first few years of the war, the British ate more fibre — and probably more vitamins too. Coincidentally, the civilian death rate actually declined, despite the psychological stresses of war and other adverse influences on the physical and social environment. It is hard to resist the belief that improved nutrition was responsible.

Richard Wilkinson believes that what happened in Britain after food rationing ended also confirms the influence of diet on death rates. Rationing, which had ensured considerable equality in food allowances throughout the population, reached its height after the war, in 1947-8, and was phased out gradually between then and the early 1950s. Thereafter, it seems, the diets of rich and poor began to diverge once more. Could this explain the spectacular widening between 1951 and 1961 of the gap in mortality rates among social classes I plus II and social classes IV plus V? Certainly those maladies which shifted most dramatically in their social distribution during the 1950s were those thought to have a predominantly dietary origin. And this was the decade when coronary heart disease, which used to be considered an affliction of the rich, became a plague of the poor.

Perinatal mortality

It is perhaps a pity that Sir John Brotherston had to deliver his masterly 1975 Galton Lecture, on inequalities in health and disease, under the auspices of the Eugenics Society. That organisation is still suspect in many people's eyes because of its historically greater devotion to the forces of nature than of nurture. In fact, Brotherston was at pains to explore and agonise over class differentials in disease in Britain. Not only does overall mortality rise regularly from social class I to social class V. These distinctions are apparent from the very outset. There are pronounced differences in perinatal mortality (still births plus deaths in the first week) among women from different backgrounds, while physical inequalities at birth continue to widen between classes as babies become children. Thus birth weights and the height and weight of school-children — measurements which are used as indices of normal healthy development — show marked and persistent inequalities in the various classes. Sir John writes:

For the most part the evidence suggests that the gaps remain as wide apart as a generation ago and in some instances the gaps may be widening. This persistence of differences and the possibility that in some instances differences may be growing greater has been a source of perplexity and disappointment to those who believe in the National Health Service as a means of bringing improved health and more equal opportunities for health within our communities.

Perinatal death rate is considered one of the prime indicators of the health of any community and the calibre of its medical services. It has received increasingly close scrutiny in recent years as, despite dazzling achievements in the realm of scientific medicine, it has often failed to improve as rapidly as expected. The United States, for example, though opening up many historic frontiers in medical research, has fallen from being world leader to fifteenth place in this measure of well being. In Britain, the Birthday Trust organised a national survey in 1958 to discover why the perinatal death rate had been stationary for the previous ten years—in contrast to the marked fall during the war years. The results showed that the rate was highest in the industrial north of England and South Wales. It was lowest in London and the south-east. Moreover, in each region the large cities had worse figures than the surrounding rural areas.

But the distribution of perinatal casualties differed. In rural parts, most of the deaths were related to difficult labour. In urban areas the excess was of deaths from prematurity and congenital malformations known to be associated with the mothers' poor health or physique. The rural women were better nourished but less able to secure skilled obstetric attention when an emergency occurred during labour. The urban women were relatively undernourished and shorter in stature, though they had a higher standard of medical care. The greater mortality in the north, too, was due to poor health and physique among the women there; those living in the south were appreciably taller, and in all areas tall women have lower perinatal mortality rates than short women. There is no reason to believe that this difference in stature is genetic; far more likely an explanation is that it too, in turn, is a result of relatively inadequate nutrition, perhaps over several generations. The basic origin must be traced not to specific physiological factors but to poverty and economic depression.

The Aberdeen experience

An outstanding instance of social perspective in the conquest of ill health is the work of Sir Dugald Baird in organising a comprehensive and progressive maternity service in Aberdeen, Scotland. In 1937 Baird was appointed to the chair of obstetrics in the city, where he established an enviably effective service and a major centre for research into perinatal mortality. Both ventures depended heavily not only on doctors with specific obstetric skills but also on experts in sociology, psychology, and epidemiology.

Baird describes his initial interest thus:

> In Aberdeen during the war it was obvious to me from clinical observation that private compared to hospital patients were much superior in their reproductive performance. In the upper social classes (I and II, corresponding roughly to private patients) women tended to marry later and were older at the time of the birth of the first child. The husband and wife had usually planned the first child and had some idea of how many they wanted. They were well informed on the facts of pregnancy and labour. The wives were on average several inches taller than hospital patients and looked much healthier. They gave birth to big babies yet difficult labour from disproportion between the baby's head and the mother's pelvis was unusual. The only disadvantage they showed was that they were older.

Using a vigorous team approach, Baird and his colleagues

set out to improve the prospects for those mothers who were *not* receiving adequate obstetric care or for one reason or another were not favourably suited to pregnancy. Expertise was certainly involved: Baird had observed the need for it while working in his previous post in Glasgow, where he found that a quarter of maternal deaths were due to haemorrhage in hospital and no transfusion service was available. But equally important were health education about nutrition and health care during pregnancy; the energetic promotion of family planning; and what for those days was a liberal attitude towards abortion. Hospital facilities were thoroughly inte-grated with the work of specialists operating in the com-munity—general practitioners, midwives and health visitors. Particular attention was paid to the best ways, times and places for deploying their skills in relation to needs.

The results won international aclaim. Despite the fact that the physique of the mothers and their social class distribution compared unfavourably with those in the south of England, the Aberdeen team managed to reduce perinatal mortality in the area to one of the lowest rates in the United Kingdom. More recently, similar principles and practices have been applied in Dundee and have shown excellent results—again in adverse social conditions.

Alas, that is not the full story. After a generation or more during which Aberdeen's obstetric services have become a model for other towns and cities throughout the world, varia-tions in perinatal mortality rates in different classes in Aberdeen remain as wide as ever. All social groups have benefited from the revolutionary policies initiated by Sir Dugald Baird, and the overall situation has improved dramati-cally. Yet marked inequalities persist.

Why? One clue comes from the work of Raymond Illsey, who analysed the movement of women in Aberdeen between social classes when they marry. He found that women who were taller and healthier moved 'upwards', while less healthy and smaller females migrated in the contrary direction. He also discovered that women who went up the social scale in this way had less perinatal mortality than those who moved down. The inevitable conclusion was that selective mating was going on, reinforcing the upper social groups with healthier recruits and having a corresponding effect in the opposite direction. As Sir John Brotherston observes:

> The dynamic processes of social mobility have the effect of concentrating at the lowest end of the social scale groups which are recruited and reinforced in a fashion which makes them most subject to morbidity and least able to make use of available resources to help themselves. It is as if we were having identified for us those for whom the traditional assumptions of the National Health Service are least effective.

Richard Titmuss was the first person to draw attention to contrasts in the use different groups in the community make of medical services. He showed that the 'middle class' in Britain were more efficient than working-class people in exploiting the National Health Service, and thus gained greater benefits from it. Such variations are bound to be reflected in morbidity statistics. And despite substantial progress towards a time when all births will take place in hospital rather than at home — formerly many of the women most in need of hospitalisation were least likely to be admitted, because of either their own decision or poor organisation — contact with maternity services still varies from one social group to another. A substantial fraction of those mothers who could benefit most still do not receive antenatal care.

Another partial explanation for the persistence of social distinctions in perinatal mortality may be the biological effects of deprivation. Dugald Baird and his colleagues have divided perinatal fatalities into two main groups: 'obstetric', in which deaths are influenced primarily by the effectiveness of obstetric care, and 'environmental', in which the causes lie in the mother's constitution and all the circumstances that have determined this. Death rates have fallen more significantly in the former category than the latter. And even in the 'obstetric' group mothers from higher social classes may profit more from competent care, because they have better general physique. Baird suggests that recent increases in perinatal death rates in some social groups in Aberdeen and elsewhere from 'environmental' causes could relate to the early upbringing of mothers during times of economic depression. Constitutional damage of this sort, he believes, could carry through into a second generation. Patterns of behaviour passed from mother to daughter could also have their influence.

Social attitudes, traditions and prejudices must play their part too. One survey showed major differences in the lifestyles of users and under-users of the maternity services. The users tended to plan their lives; the under-users were 'crisis-motivated'. There is also a sizeable lag, when health services are reorganised, before people become aware of the fact and begin to respond. Meanwhile, longstanding habits of infant care and hygiene persist. Perhaps most clear-cut is the example of a working-class mother with several children who may be unwilling, or find it extremely difficult, to enter hospital for her confinement.

Finally, there remains the stark fact that, despite everything achieved in a city like Aberdeen, high-quality medical attention is not equally accessible across the community. A survey by Ann Cartwright published in 1964 showed that in predominantly working-class areas in Britain 80 per cent of doctors' surgeries dated from before 1900, whereas less than half of those in middle-class areas had been built before that year, and a quarter had been constructed since 1945 — compared with five per cent in working class districts. More of the general practitioners in middle-class areas had lists of less than 2,000 patients and fewer had lists of over 2,500. Nearly twice as many possessed higher qualifications. More had access to specialised X-ray facilities and nearly five times as many had access to physiotherapy. Twice the proportion held hospital appointments or had hospital beds into which they could admit their own patients. All of this, too, in a country with a

National Health Service founded upon the principle that medical care should be available equally to everyone in the community irrespective of social or financial status. Such irregularities make themselves felt even more forcibly in the morbidity statistics of a country like the United States, whose medical facilities are largely the product of market forces.

We have moved a considerable way, from myopic pre-occupation with specific disease entities to a position where we see that the real shape of man's morbidity and mortality is discernible only from a social vantage point. The career of Sir Dugald Baird, one of the most far-seeing medical men of recent years, illustrates the change vividly. When he began work as a young doctor, deaths of mothers in childbirth were so common as to dominate the practice of obstetrics. Child-bed fever, in those pre-antibiotic days, was still a serious hazard. Amidst overwhelming maternal and infant mortality, perinatal fatalities were hardly considered. But despite all that, the great contrast between childbearing in the upper social classes and in slum dwellers set Baird thinking and led to his lasting interest in the social aspects of disease. As a pioneer he had to face considerable hostility and resistance before others began to see the point of his evangelising.

Urbanisation and disease

Today, the World Health Organisation, whose most dramatic achievements in the past have been in vanquishing specific pathogens such as the smallpox virus, is extending greatly its concern for the social ramifications of disease. One topic high-lighted in its recent report *Promoting Health in the Human Environment* is urbanisation and the growth of cities:

Immigrants tend to move into the deteriorating central quarters of cheap lodging houses, which typically adjoin bleak industrial sites and office blocks vacated nightly. This combination of slums, high mobility, impersonality, and industrial squalor provides the necessary social and physical conditions in which disease and hopeless misery multiply, and hence psychological and social disorders as well . . . In some cities the major problem might be the plight of unassimilated, starving immigrants; in others, disease-ridden slums; and yet in others, the task of organising and implementing health services in the face of economic, educational and political obstacles.

Several epidemiological surveys have confirmed that the prevalence of both mental and organic disease in cities reflects their ecological pattern. Thus psychiatric illness, together with alcoholism and drug abuse, thrive in areas where the 'social cement' is weakened because people have become alienated from social and cultural forces. Schizophrenic, neurotic and psychopathic disorders are unusually common in both impoverished and socially disorganised districts. Suicide has a different distribution. Case studies have revealed that, while individuals committing or attempting suicide have significantly fewer ties with their family, neighbourhood or occupational or religious groups, their social status (as defined by class and education) tends to be higher. Alienation and poverty do not necessarily go together.

The WHO report points out that less psychologically stable people often fail socially and may therefore accumulate in the more deteriorated districts of the cities. Harsh social conditions—lack of space, privacy, and basic amenities; long working hours; noise—can also contribute to stress and thus the development of psychosomatic conditions such as peptic ulcer. But sometimes an impoverished environment has the opposite effect; poverty, loneliness, and boring work may lead to apathy and depression. The report concludes:

Many of the untoward effects on health and social problems of the poor, the aged, and the ethnic minorities are therefore related to the extent to which they are socially isolated. Well-intentioned efforts to improve the physical environment can have unhappy consequences when authorities fail to recognise this. Thus urban rehousing projects that break up well-knit neighbourhoods and kinship groups can lead to impairment of the social and emotional life of the new residents. Similarly, the consensus is that the elderly and mothers with young families find that high-rise flats make uncongenial homes and are no substitute for the greater intimacy of houses along the street.

But urbanisation does not always presage a deterioration in community health, even in developing countries. That is clear from a study of the population in a mining area in Sierra Leone, carried out by Dr A. R. Mills. He found that people living in the new industrial town of Lunsar in the northern province of the country were fitter than those in the surrounding villages — even though the town was more crowded. Dr Mills concluded that, with careful planning, well-designed factories and homes, and high standards of medical care and public hygiene, industrialisation in developing countries need not lead to the miseries which were so common in the eighteenth and nineteenth centuries in Britain.

Poverty and mobility

'Socioeconomic stress' is another factor identified by the WHO report. Poverty causes illness by depriving people of basic needs of shelter, hygiene, and adequate nutrition, and thus both increases their exposure to infections and makes them more vulnerable to them. It also means that they are less likely to have access to health services and — perhaps most important — it debilitates people, predisposes them to fatigue and apathy, and engenders frustration and despair. The effects of poverty on health seem to depend on the context within which the poverty is experienced. Thus poverty which is imposed suddenly as a result of ill fortune may be much harder to bear than that into which a person has been born. This is particularly true in communities that have a tradition of mutual support and shared adversity. Suicide statistics support this idea. During the 1930s economic depression in Britain, the lowest suicide rates were among the poorest sectors of the population. They were the only classes in which suicide did not increase during that period. The more affluent classes had the highest rates ever recorded. Similarly, suicide and attempted suicide are particularly common among people who have lost their job (for reasons other than illness).

Social mobility has its effects on disease too. This is seen most strikingly in countries changing from a rural to an industrial society, when migrant labour poses a problem. In these circumstances, when workers move vast distances with their families to seek work, the children are often neglected and housing is often grossly inadequate. Malnutrition is common. But if the male travels alone in search of employment he loses contact with his family. The children suffer by his absence, and he may become promiscuous, which can help spread venereal disease.

Again, suicide is an accurate measure of mental well-being. Both migrants and immigrants have higher suicide rates than the native born, and the effect is most pronounced in the two years following a move. They are also more prone to mental disorder. The WHO report cites a survey showing that immigrants from rural districts into cities had greater mortality from coronary heart disease than those born in a city. At all ages, cardiovascular death rates among persons of foreign birth were above those of their compatriots in the country of origin. Hypertension was more common in tribal Africans who moved into an industrial society, while factory workers who came from rural areas had worse records for absenteeism than had the urbanised workers. It could be that people who elect to emigrate are simply a more vulnerable group, but there is good evidence to the contrary. The observed effects appear to be real results of immigration and migration.

Man's maladjustment

Dr Stephen Boyden has outlined two contrasting philosophies which underly society's attempts to cope with 'biological maladjustments' which manifest themselves as disease. One, the corrective approach, attempts to remove the fundamental causes of such maladjustments. The other, the antidotal method, is dedicated to the tactic of treating the symptoms or other effects of disease — by using specific therapies. We have developed maladjustments because our environment has altered much more rapidly than we have been able to adapt through biological evolution. The environmental changes range from increases in the background radiation to which we expose ourselves to the replacement of work as a social activity by impersonal mass-production. Most of them are likely to encourage the development of disease.

A curious example of the way scientific man has responded to his own maladjustment concerns blood pressure. For many years, textbooks have explained that after the age of twenty years blood pressure gradually rises, even in healthy people. In fact, studies in New Guinea and elsewhere have now established that blood pressure does not necessarily increase with advancing years in people living in simple, non-westernised societies. The phenomenon we have described as normal is not normal at all, but stems from an adverse environment.

There is, it seems, a mismatch between modern medicine, founded securely on the notion that illnesses are caused by viruses and other specifically offensive agents, and the 'diseases of civilisation', such as coronary heart trouble, which arise from biological maladjustment. In drawing attention to this disparity, Boyden neither advocates a return to the primeval state nor argues that our hunter-gatherer ancestors were 'better off' in general than we are. He does insist that many of the illnesses and ailments in modern society are the consequence of deviations in life conditions and lifestyle and they are not therefore inevitable aspects of human life. They are not unavoidable.

Malaria and behaviour

Consideration of social environment is helpful not only in understanding certain diseases but also in trying to combat them. Malaria is one example. After decades on the receiving end of conventional warfare, this pestilence is now thwarting man's best endeavours once more. Each year over a million children die of the disease in Africa alone. Many millions of victims are condemned each year to a life of debility and apathy. New ideas are necessary to aid the fight, and one man who has put forward a strategy based on sociology rather than specific therapy is Professor David Gillett. He argues that the traditional, neat picture of infectious disease, centred solely on parasites and their vectors as *the* enemy and as *the* weak link where the transmission chain can be broken, has had undue influence. So, while throwing massive resources into anti-mosquito campaigns, we have largely neglected the other component in the system: man himself. Spreading oil on water where mosquitoes breed and spraying DDT on house walls, Gillett suggests, will not make malaria disappear. We have deceived ourselves if we believe otherwise. Such strategems and modern, increasingly sophisticated probes into the ultrastructure, serology, genetics, and physiology of parasites and their vectors should not be abandoned overnight. But if substantial practical progress is to be achieved they must be supplemented by a new, man-oriented approach.

David Gillett's proposal rests on treating human behaviour as at least as important as the biology of the mosquito. Historically, malaria and other insect-borne diseases have been eradicated in many areas before modern insecticides and drugs became available. Self-help, local motivation and organisation have often been crucial. The alternative situation, however, in which 'a poverty-stricken peasantry sits back to await treatment by some benevolent but equally poverty-stricken government' is all too common today. Technology based on the simplistic premise of specific aetiology is inappropriate, to say the least, in such circumstances.

How, then, to fire communities and individuals with the need for action and vigilance, so that drugs and mosquito nets *are* properly used and public exhortations seem genuinely, personally important rather than boring instructions handed out by well-meaning officials? Professor Gillett's approach would be to use the most potent of public relations techniques, not conventional health education:

Mosquitoes mean misery; malaria leads to poverty; health means success, success in business and success with the other sex. Mosquitoes lead to deformity to sterility, to weakness and impotence. These are the messages that must be indirectly but subtly conveyed, mainly by example: Antonio, vigorous and virile, succeeds in trade, in politics, and with women, but Yakabo, riddled with parasitic disease, fails in almost all that he sets out to do. The mosquito net and the anti-malaria pill must replace the dangling cigarette as the symbol of status and success.

Professor Gillett's point is well taken. The challenge of health propaganda is to make it individually, personally stimulating. The problem is all the greater when the aim is to urge the prevention, rather than treatment, of disease, which we shall be considering in the next chapter. Wonder drugs hit the headlines, as do heart transplants, brain surgery, and kidney machines. These are all specific measures to combat specific diseases, the exciting products of medical science. In comparison, eating nutritious food, cleaner living, giving up smoking, and avoiding undue stress amount to a strikingly uninteresting catalogue of virtue. Financial inducements and penalties may help us to take notice of such injunctions. But in the end, as the American experience with prohibition showed, what counts is what we as individuals deem to be reasonable and in our own interests.

7
Prevent or cure?

Even its most stringent opponents concede that Britain's National Health Service is competent in dealing with serious, acute disease. In converting sick persons into healthy ones by applying specific correctives, whether of chemotherapy or surgery, the NHS has an international reputation. But, compared with the mass of morbidity in the community, cases of fulminating meningitis (a rapidly worsening, potentially fatal brain infection, requiring the speedy administration of antibiotics) or mitral stenosis (narrowing of the orifice of the heart's mitral valve, needing sophisticated surgery) are few and far between. So one of the two main medical criticisms of the NHS is that it is overspecialised, hospital- rather than community-oriented, and insensitive to the great burden of chronic ill health which numerically and personally is vastly more significant than rare emergencies, traumas, and acute episodes. The second allegation is that the NHS is really an Ill Health Service, organised to cope with disease rather than to foster health. But that criticism, to which we turn in this chapter, is not peculiar to the NHS. It applies just as forcibly in other Western countries and highlights a flaw that can be traced to the exaggerated dominance of specific aetiology in the development of modern medicine.

The story of roughage

Fibre provides an excellent example. The evolution of

nutritional science and dietetics was directed by successive attempts to pinpoint the physiological roles of particular chemical constituents in food. First came the recognition of the need for specific vitamins (and trace elements), absence of which led to characteristic diseases. Then, using laboratory paraphernalia to measure the energy value of different nutrients, scientists worked out human food requirements with increasing precision. Minimum levels of fat, carbohydrate and especially protein were computed, on the basis that the body functions like a machine with standard demands for these building materials and energy sources. This approach is admirably summarised in the following passage by Professor W. D. Halliburton from the book *Physiology and National Needs*, published in 1919:

> In order to explain the word nutrition we may roughly compare the body to a steam-engine. To maintain this in running order it is necessary (1) to supply it with fuel, and (2) to keep it in repair. The burning of the fuel gives rise to heat and also generates the work which it is the object of the engine to accomplish... A nutritious diet is one which is able to repair tissue waste and provide the requisite amount of energy.

Amidst all of this quantification fibre was overlooked. Indeed, the objectives of modern milling are to obliterate it as completely as possible from flour. First, the endosperm (the storage material of the wheat germ, which contains the bulk of the starch) is separated from the bran and germ. This is done to obtain flour that has no specks of bran and which contains no indigestible residue. The second aim is to reduce as much of the endosperm as possible to flour, so as to gain the best possible 'extraction rate'. Milling removes some nutrients, but the necessary vitamins and minerals, in a state of high purity, are replaced. Most countries now have statutory minimal levels of two of the B group vitamins and iron. Flour must be reinforced with these constituents to agreed levels. Chalk is usually incorporated too, as a means of preventing calcium deficiency in the population. Thus modern flour is chemically defined, and designed to be totally digestible, each constituent having a specific role to play in maintaining the bodily engine.

Only recently have we realised that removal of bran from flour was followed historically by considerable increases in the prevalence of appendicitis and diverticulitis. These conditions, together with colon cancer and constipation, are rare in rural Africa and Asia to this day, but become common as communities change to a Western diet. Diverticular disease and its associated bowel cancer were both virtually unknown in Britain in 1900. Regardless of ethnic origin, when people change to a diet containing refined flour and sugar these diseases appear within a generation. With the advance of nutritional science based on the concept of specific nutrients 'indigestible' became a dirty word, but now we are beginning to recognise that to maintain health our diet should contain a sizeable proportion of such undefined, non-specific, chemically useless roughage. By consuming adequate amounts of fibre, we could, it seems, prevent many of those diseases which currently devour enormous medical resources when they have to be dealt with surgically.

Avoidable deaths

So too with most of the afflictions causing most of the morbidity in modern Western societies. Of the ten leading causes of death from disease in the United States in 1974, the majority were conditions for which we already have either preventive measures or enough basic knowledge to suggest that research into prevention would pay off.

Cardiovascular disease (39 per cent of total deaths in 1974) includes one condition, rheumatic heart disease, that can be prevented by swift antibiotic treatment of the streptococcal infection that is originally responsible. Most of the cases in this category, however, are of coronary disease. Here the thrust of contemporary medical practice is towards means of dealing with emergencies: intensive care units and special mobile ambulances for the victims of heart attacks; digitalis and diuretics for heart failure; and the surgical replacement of damaged valves, arteries and even — in some enthusiastic centres — whole hearts. Yet we know (see p. 80) that regular exercise, avoidance of smoking, and other aspects of lifestyle have a measurable influence overall in reducing the likelihood of heart attack. The only weakness of such measures is that their application rests on will-power and their value, for any one individual, is shrouded in uncertainty. The man who can speak of 'my tablets' or 'my operation' can have no solid guarantee that his morning job or indecision to give up cigarette smoking will have a tangible effect on his cardiovascular future.

Cancer (19 per cent of deaths) is the other major category where treatment — by surgery, radiation, and drugs — remains our principal means of combat. As we shall see, however (p. 180), there are prospects that we could forestall the appearance of a considerable proportion of malignant tumours in the first place by reducing exposure to environmental and dietary hazards. The pattern for such evasive action has already been established for asbestos.

Kidney disease (10.4 per cent of deaths) comprises two main conditions, both of which can precipitate chronic failure of the organ. Transplantation, or frequent dialysis in which the patient's blood is cleansed by being routed through an artificial kidney machine, are the mainstays of management. But swift attention to, or prevention of, the infections leading to renal failure can prevent many of these fatal failures. Even more important for the future is the prospect of curbing the urinary tract infections which usually precede kidney infection — but which usually go undetected (see p. 175).

Cerebrovascular diseases (11 per cent of deaths), principally strokes, remain a challenge to preventive medicine. Compared with coronary disease, there is less direct evidence that people can avoid such catastrophes by living more sensible lives. But, given that most strokes are associated with atherosclerosis or hypertension (a few result from congenitally weak blood vessels in the brain), there is a basis for believing in the benefit of similar measures. This is one field where more research is required.

Pulmonary disease (4.5 per cent of deaths) includes a range of maladies, from chronic bronchitis to influenza. Bronchitis is certainly avoidable: its rarity among the non-smoking well off attests to that. In principle, it should never reach the stage where medical practitioners have to douse their patients in antibiotics every winter to keep it under control. Other forms of chronic obstructive lung disease, such as pneumoconiosis among miners, are largely occupational and may be thwarted by minimising workers' exposure to fine dusts: Influenza is a greater problem: there is no reason to think that a virulent virus like that which ravaged the world in 1918-19 should not emerge again. Assuming that Western man will continue to live in comparatively crowded conditions, unlike his hunter-gatherer ancestors for whom infectious disease was much less bothersome, the chief stratagem for prevention is the use of vaccines. A magic bullet to treat influenza seems an unlikely proposition.

Diabetes (1.9 per cent of deaths) provides a crystal-clear example of specific aetiology at work: provision of a particular hormone, insulin, brings the disease under control. It could, in time, also become a model for preventive medicine. Many cases result from obesity. By avoiding getting fat, therefore, we reduce our chances of becoming diabetic. But there is also evidence (see p. 168) that the condition may be avoided altogether simply by dispensing with the vast quantities of sugar with which we now batter our metabolism.

Cirrhosis of the liver (1.8 per cent of deaths) can be evaded by renouncing alcohol. All but a vanishingly small number of cases are caused by heavy drinking over a long period of time. Cirrhosis, like alcoholism, is increasing in most Western societies. Both conditions are unquestionably avoidable.

Perinatal disease (1.5 per cent of deaths) includes some

conditions, like hyaline disease of the newborn (a failure of the lungs to begin working properly), for which there is no specific therapy. But the enormous differences in perinatal mortality rates in different countries show that much can be done to reduce these deaths. The answers lie in nutrition, in environment, and in antenatal and obstetric care.

Congenital malformations and deficiencies (0.7 per cent of deaths) are afflictions towards which medical opinion has turned around sharply already in favour of prevention. In the past, such defects as spina bifida posed challenges to surgical expertise, and great skills have been developed with which to reduce handicap as far as possible and give the victims useful life. Today, the trend is towards methods of identifying severe congenital abnormalities in the growing foetus, so that parents can be offered the choice of abortion.

Peptic ulcers (those in the region of the stomach and the duodenum, responsible for 0.5 per cent of deaths) seem to be a peculiar scourge of 'civilisation'. A variety of drugs and surgical treatments are available, but avoidance of the stress, strain, smoking, and silly eating habits known to encourage ulceration is a sounder approach.

Painless prevention

A few years ago Dr N. B. Belloc and Dr L. Breslow conducted an intriguing survey in which, instead of seeking to identify specific tactics helpful in warding off distinct illnesses, they identified a lifestyle that appeared to engender good health. After studying nearly 7,000 adults over five and a half years, they found that life expectancy and health were related significantly to seven basic habits. These were: taking three meals a day at regular times, with no snacks in between; eating breakfast every day; exercising moderately two or three times a week; having adequate sleep (seven or eight hours each night); not smoking; maintaining a modest weight; and consuming no alcohol or taking it only in moderation. Drs Belloc and

Breslow calculated that the remaining life expectancy of a 45-year-old man who followed at most three of these injunctions was 21.6 years, while that for a man following six or seven of them was 33.1 years. Thus relatively simple changes in an individual's way of life may be sufficient to add over a decade to his life.

In effect, the inactive, overweight man who is a heavy smoker and drinker and takes irregular meals and sleep is not just shortening his lifespan. He is in a real sense accelerating parts of his own ageing process. Dr Breslow found that the 'health status' of those who practised all seven of his healthy habits was similar to that of men thirty years younger who observed none of them. Up to 80 per cent of deaths from cardiovascular disease and cancer are premature, in that they occur in relatively young people and are brought on by their own abuses. Overweight is a particularly potent influence for ill health. An estimated 16 per cent of Americans under 30 are obese, and 40 per cent of the total population (80 million people) are at least 20 lbs above the ideal weight for their height, sex, and age. More than 30 per cent of men between 50 and 59 years are 20 per cent overweight, and 60 per cent are at least 10 per cent over.

The consequences are well documented. One of the largest ever surveys of heart disease, carried out in Framingham, Massachusetts, indicated that each 10 per cent weight reduction by men 35-55 years of age would lead to a 20 per cent decrease in the incidence of coronary disease. A 10 per cent rise in weight would result in a 30 per cent increase in the condition. Moreover, obesity encourages innumerable maladies other than heart trouble. They include liver and gall bladder disease; degenerative arthritis of the hips, knees, and ankles; and many more.

At the other end of the scale is malnutrition, with its own associated diseases. This is an overwhelming problem in the Third World (see p. 189). But 26 million Americans (11 million of whom receive no federal food assistance) also live below the federally defined poverty level—a level that does not support an adequate diet.

Disparities thus persist between vast investment in curative medicine and minimal spending on measures of avoidance. Of a total expenditure on medicine in the United States of 120 billion dollars per annum, at most 2½ per cent goes to disease prevention and control. A mere half a per cent is for health education and for action to improve the organisation and delivery of health services. The federal budget for environmental health research is about a quarter of one per cent of total medical expenditure. Yet, as Dr John Knowles, president of the Rockefeller Foundation, puts it:

If no one smoked cigarettes or consumed alcohol and everyone exercised regularly, maintained optimal weight on a low-fat, low refined-carbohydrate, high fibre-content diet, reduced stress by simplifying their lives, obtained adequate rest and recreation, understood the needs of infants and children for the proper nutrition and nurturing of their intellectual and effective development, had available to them and would use genetic counselling and selective abortion, drank fluoridated water, followed the doctor's orders for medications and self-care once disease was detected, and used available health services at the appropriate time for screening examinations and health education-preventive medicine programs, the savings to the country would be mammoth in terms of millions of dollars, a vast reduction in human misery, and an attendant marked improvement in the quality of life.

Dr Knowles believes that the next major advances in the health of the American people will be determined not by frontier science but by 'what the individual is willing to do for himself and for society-at-large'. Individuals should take action in three ways: by adopting Belloc and Breslow's seven golden rules, by encouraging their children in the same direction, and by participating actively in public affairs to reduce environmental hazards and further the cause of preventive medicine. On public policy, Knowles argues that health education should be integrated much more fully into the school system, with an emphasis on what individuals can do for themselves. Taxes on cigarettes and spirits should be increased considerably, and selective screening and counselling services should be developed to identify and check latent ill health. 'The health of human beings is determined by their behaviour, their food, and the nature of the environment,' Knowles concludes. 'Over 99 per cent of us are born healthy and suffer premature death and disability only as a result of personal misbehaviour and environmental conditions.'

The economic arguments

Dr Knowles is on sure ground when he pins most of his hopes on individuals rather than on confidence that the medical establishment will shift its traditional stance massively away from specific therapies and towards preventive policies. The interest that has grown up in recent years in the positive fostering of health has come largely from the environmentalists and advocates of alternative lifestyles rather than from doctors or governments. The American figures for expenditure on curative as against preventive medicine are reflected in Britain, for example, where, in 1972 a journal, *Prevent*, was launched to promote this approach but failed due to lack of support. Only in 1976 did the Department of Health and Social Security in the United Kingdom take its first tangible steps in this direction. It did so by issuing as a consultative document, the report *Prevention and Health: Everybody's Business.*

Introducing the report, Mrs Barbara Castle and her colleagues had this to say: 'It is at least possible that in the absence of unforeseen and economical new methods of treatment, curative medicine may be increasingly subject to the law of diminishing returns. Accordingly we believe that the time has come for a re-appraisal of the possibilities inherent in prevention.' The immediate stimulus for the document was the reorganisation of Britain's Health Service in 1974, when moves were made, including the setting up of 'community health councils', to foster greater collaboration between doctors and other health workers, thereby emphasising the social context of medicine. Disease prevention, in the form of immunisation programmes and food inspection, was formerly the concern almost solely of the local authorities. *Prevention and Health* is a recognition of the fact that this approach should permeate and inform all aspects of the health services.

It is also relevant that the report was produced at a time of unusually severe economic ill health. The notion that prevention can be much cheaper than cure carries correspondingly greater force than before. A week in a typical hospital bed in Britain now costs an average of nearly £150, so the avoidable admissions, for lung cancer, chronic bronchitis, depression, and a string of other conditions, could save the country a considerable amount of money.

The financial arguments surrounding preventive medicine are, of course, complex. Setting aside the loss of tax to the government (and of revenue to the manufacturers) when someone gives up smoking and thereby escapes lung cancer, it can also be argued that the apparent saving to the community in not having to provide for his or her treatment is more apparent than real. Instead of dying in their early forties, such people may live to reach an age at which they become dependent on public funds. They may well develop, and eventually die of, other chronic conditions that require medical attention, also at public expense. Against this, however, is the fact that the forestalling of a fatal illness does not simply avert early death; it also ensures that a person carries on an active life during which, up to retirement perhaps, he or she is earning money. Moreover, even if prevention only postpones for some years the time when the costs of medical care are incurred, this has an economic value that can be substantial.

Down's syndrome (mongolism) may now be detected long before birth using a technique known as amniocentesis to collect some of the fluid surrounding the foetus. Cells in the liquid are then examined in the laboratory for the characteristic signs of chromosome abnormality and the foetus may then be aborted. The current cost of a single test in Britain is £80. In purely economic terms, this prenatal screening appears prudent. Many more mongol children now survive infancy. The cost of keeping a person in a hospital for the mentally handicapped is about £2,000 per year, while that of special education is approximately £1,000 a year. On such figures, it seems that for mothers aged over forty the costs to society of caring for those affected — as children and as adults — would exceed that of a screening programme. In the case of younger mothers, however, who are much less likely to produce a foetus affected in this way, the economic advantages of amniocentesis are less certain. Preventive screening should be used not indiscriminately but with judgement.

These examples illustrate two alternative strategies of preventive medicine. The first is to discourage the emergence of disease by adjusting the way we live. Alternatively, ill health and latent ill health can be identified by screening at an early stage and dealt with accordingly. Both contrast with the administration of specific panaceas for overt maladies — the principle upon which orthodox Western medicine is built. It is illuminating to compare these approaches in the case of a single condition: diabetes.

Dealing with diabetes

Dr G. D. Campbell, of the Durban Diabetes Study Project in South Africa, believes that we are all pre-diabetics. What turns some of us into clinical specimens of the disease is our unnatural intake of purified sugar (sucrose), which is tolerable by some but potentially lethal to others. Campbell's views are based almost entirely on epidemiology and studies of diet. They gain little from scientific work in the laboratory. While diabetes is a disease of great antiquity — Ayurvedic writers described it 3,500 years ago as 'holy urine' (because of the vast amount of sugar that appears in a diabetic's water) — it appears to have been uncommon. That meticulous observer and recorder Hippocrates never described a single case. Diabetes is rare in rural peasants but prevalent in people of the same stock who have migrated into an urban environment. And in 1929 Dr Frederick Banting observed that sugar plantation owners who ate large quantities of refined sugar had a much higher frequency of diabetes than the cane cutters who got their sugar by chewing cane. While diabetes has been described as one of the 'diseases of urbanisation', it is also common among rural peoples who are sufficiently affluent to be able to afford a diet rich in sugar and other refined carbohydrates.

Diabetes is one of those diseases which disappear at times when food is scarce or severely rationed. This was apparent during the Siege of Paris in 1871, and again in occupied Europe and in Germany towards the end of the Second World War. Observations in animals afford further evidence. Diabetes is some six times more frequent in the carbohydrate-oriented domestic cat than in the domestic dog with its preference for protein.

What counts seems to be not the quantity of calories but their quality. Dr Campbell, for example, found that sugar cane cutters on the north coast of Natal who had a high daily consumption of 5,000 - 6,000 calories, but who obtained most of their sugar by chewing sugar cane, never developed diabetes. And a comparison in 1959 of the diets of Zulus in rural areas (where there was no diabetes) and urban parts (where the disease was common) showed that calorie intake was actually slightly greater in the rural people. Carbohydrate constituted 55 per cent of the total in both groups, but the town dwellers took this in a refined condition — chiefly sugar, white bread, and foods sweetened with sugar. In the country, carbohydrate was consumed largely in the form of home-pounded cereals. The picture has changed dramatically since that time, as sugar eating has increased in rural areas following energetic promotion and advertising. The high prevalence of diabetes in some Red Indian tribes is also associated with a low-calorie diet —

but one in which a substantial proportion of those calories come as refined carbohydrate.

Seventy pounds of sugar per head per annum seems to be the figure that divides countries where diabetes is common from those in which the disease is a rarity. This accords with studies by Professor J. A. Tulloch in various tropical countries, and also with the results of the fall in sugar consumption during wartime. The other significant statistic is 20 per cent. Where the intake of calories as sugar exceeds this value diabetes is prevalent even among people on a low total calorie diet.

Diabetes thus seems to be a condition that is determined overwhelmingly via food — and, in turn, by social customs and eating habits. What of genetic factors? At one time, diabetics were advised not to marry one another, as this was thought to increase the likelihood of diabetes in the child and increase the frequency of genes predisposing to the condition. The wisdom of this advice is now in serious doubt. Genetic influences in the emergence of diabetes seem to have been grossly exaggerated. Many apparently hereditary effects may in fact have resulted from learning eating habits.

Dr Campbell's methods of dealing with diabetes would consist of a programme of health education together with economic and political pressures to reduce the per capita sugar intake in all countries to the figure of 70 lb. per annum. Synthetic sweeteners should be made available, and the World Health Organisation should seek to curb the highly slanted advertisements issued, especially in developing countries, to promote sucrose consumption. Sugar should be diverted into industrial use, as a raw material for producing motor fuels and other synthetics, and be converted by microorganisms into protein for animal fodder. Sugar beet production, which is wasteful in the use of sunlight in temperate climates, should be ended and the acreages turned over to other food crops.

A totally different approach to the disease is to scrutinise apparently healthy people for signs of latent diabetes so that they can be given drugs to reduce their blood sugar or be advised to adjust their diet accordingly. This is only one of many tests that are used in 'multiphasic screening', a system pioneered in the United States by the Kaiser-Permanente Medical Foundation, in which fit persons are examined for indications of incipient ill health. X-rays, blood tests, and even personality questionnaires are employed to weed out individuals who may, without knowing it, be in need of advice or treatment. The test for 'hidden' diabetes is typical.

A simple analysis for sugar in the urine has long been employed to identify diabetics and pre-diabetics. It is, for example, a routine measure used on recruits to the armed forces, hospital patients, applicants for life insurance, and many job candidates. A more sophisticated and sensitive tool is a test of the quantity of sugar in a person's bloodstream a measured time after he has taken a standard dose of sugar by mouth. Whereas urine examination brings to light some early diabetics, it does not give conclusive results. There may be 'false positives' and more importantly 'false negatives', people who are suffering from mild diabetes but do not have sugar in their urine when tested.

Professor Harry Keen, from Guy's Hospital, London, calculates that a survey of the entire UK population for diabetes using a simple urine analysis would probably yield between 10 and 20 per cent of positive results. These people should then be examined again with the more sophisticated (and more expensive) blood test. About 2 per cent of the initial group, he estimates, may finally come under medical care and require drug treatment. The expense of such an exercise has to be set against 'the potential economic savings, the cost of hospital beds and medical manpower, of absence from work through illness, and the loss of productive efficiency. These can hardly be guessed at at present, and do not take into account the mitigation of personal suffering, on which only the individual can set a price.'

One of the problems of screening is that it can create a vast amount of work for the medical profession. That was precisely what happened when Professor Keen and his colleagues conducted a diabetic survey in 1962 in the town of Bedford. They uncovered so many cases of the disease that the local clinic could not cope with them. Even if they had surveyed the population more slowly, they would still have found more diabetics than could have been dealt with easily by the hard-pressed medical manpower in the town. Another objection to mass screening for diabetes is that the benefits to be derived from early care of people not aware of their condition are not incontestably certain. Clearly, any pathological process is more likely to be reversible in its early stages than later on. There is evidence that individuals with mild diabetes who are identified and whose blood sugar is brought down by dieting or drug treatment do better in the long run than those who go undetected. But the results are not black and white. Stopping the disease from ever appearing — as Dr Campbell advocates — remains a better option than preventing it from developing. Both are preferable to the *laissez-faire* approach of awaiting the evolution of florid diabetes before administering the appropriate hormone.

The hidden iceberg

As a half-way house between outright prevention of disease by healthy living and the more conventional attitude of specific therapy for established afflictions, mass screening has achieved undoubted successes. The conquest of pulmonary tuberculosis in the United States and Europe owed as much to X-ray campaigns as it did to streptomycin and the other wonder drugs used to defeat the tubercle bacillus. Mass radiography was employed to excellent effect before these antibiotics were even discovered. Similarly, the schedule of care designed to detect irregularities during pregnancy has paid handsome dividends. The existence of a 'clinical iceberg' of undetected disease, shown by surveys in many different countries, implies that very much more could be done. One study conducted in an average general practice in the United Kingdom revealed 30 men and 131 women with high blood pressure. The condition of only 8 of the men and 24 of the women was already known to this doctor. There were 140 urinary tract infections in women, only 25 of them detected previously. Corresponding figures revealed for the first time many cases of rheumatoid arthritis, glaucoma, cervical cancer, and psychiatric abnormalities.

Why does the iceberg exist? The theory of specific aetiology must bear a large part of the blame. Medical services generally are geared to dealing with clear symptoms and discrete complaints. Doctors and indeed other sectors of the medical care organisation give priority to patients with overt disease rather than to apparently healthy people or those with vague, minimal illness. Many of the latter do not wish to bother their doctors anyway — and in a country like the United States they may also be inhibited financially from doing so. One investigation in Britain showed that even people with indications of diabetes hesitated before asking advice; 48 per cent tolerated daily symptoms for four months before approaching their medical practitioner, and 20 per cent waited over a year.

One of the outstanding successes of mass screening in recent years has come from the early diagnosis of cervical cancer. Efficiently applied, cervical cytology — the microscopic examination of cells from the neck of the womb — can turn a 70 per cent mortality into a 90 - 100 per cent cure. This form of cancer is accessible, for both the examination of tissue and subsequent treatment. The clearest evidence of the benefits of screening comes from the province of British Columbia, where a cytology laboratory was first established in 1949. Over the period 1955 - 66, during which about two-thirds of the female population was tested one or more times, the prevalence of clinical carcinoma declined by 53 per cent. The fall in incidence for the sector of the population that was screened was 85 per cent — a figure that should approach 100 per cent if errors can be reduced and if women are examined annually. The consequences of early detection are clear: in British Columbia, where the screening rate is probably the highest in the world, deaths from the disease have dropped from 15 to 7 per 100,000 women.

Cervical cytology is clearly worthwhile—though here again many tumours could be prevented from developing in the first place. Cancer of the cervix is commoner among women from an unfavourable socioeconomic background, among those who have had many sexual partners beginning at an early age, and those who have been infected with a herpes virus that is transmitted sexually. Celibate women are at very low risk. Personal hygiene also seems to be important in minimising the chances of the disease developing.

Screening for breast cancer is more controversial. Clinical examination (often beginning with self-examination for lumps) combined with the X-ray technique known as mamography reveals breast tumours at an early stage, though the evidence that detection followed by treatment can reduce mortality is less than spectacular. The only extensive study yet reported, conducted under the auspices of the Health Insurance Plan of Greater New York, showed some benefit. During a seven-year follow-up period, there were a third fewer deaths among 30,000 women who had been offered four examinations at yearly intervals than among a comparable group who were not offered screening. This compares with the halving of deaths from cervical cancer in British Columbia, and realistic hopes for even better results. One should be cautious about assuming that dramatic results could be achieved by nationwide screening projects in the case of breast cancer. And the costs would be considerable.

This is one of the problems tackled in *Prevention and Health*, a document which expresses faith in the practice of preventive medicine, coupled with anxiety about whether Britain can afford it. One nuisance about screening for breast cancer is that it yields at least five false positives for every tumour detected. Each of these requires further investigation—a surgical biopsy and laboratory investigation—which throws an additional load on the corresponding services. Moreover, the Health Insurance Plan study demonstrated a definite reduction in mortality only among women in their fifties. There are some 3.5 million women in Britain of that age.

Assuming a response rate of 60 per cent, a programme of annual screening would require 2.1 million tests, and the number of cancers detected would be around 3,000. There would also be some 15,000 biopsies on false positive cases. Thus a national screening programme only for women between 50 and 60 would require about £20-30 millions per annum. The DHSS calculates that the cost per life prolonged would be £8,000.

There are two possible responses to this situation. One is to plough greater resources into research towards improved tests, which would eliminate false positives and identify those women for whom regular screening is particularly worthwhile. The other is to turn again to the environmental and dietary origins of cancer (see p. 180), with a view to eliminating the carcinogens responsible for minimising exposure to them.

The commonest bacterial infection known is that of the urinary tract. It is often persistent, and even when eliminated tends to recur. Many studies have shown that it is a serious cause of morbidity and mortality in the community—both directly, and indirectly by triggering infection of the kidney, which can lead to chronic renal failure. The control of urinary infection, particularly in women, is thus an urgent problem. It could undoubtedly be dealt with by an efficient screening programme. The infections are typically mixed—no specific pathogens are involved—and the tests for demonstrating the presence of bacteria are elementary.

Pregnancy is a time of special risk. A pregnant woman can have bacteria in her urine without being conscious of the fact, and this can become a kidney infection and in turn precipitate acute renal failure. The same may happen in people other than pregnant women, particularly those whose natural resistance is impaired because of poor nutrition or other causes. The dangers that symptomless, chronic urinary tract infection can produce an equally symptom-free infection of the kidney are illustrated by one survey which showed that in one in four of people unaware of their urinary condition the kidneys were also affected. Moreover, chronic kidney infection is now thought to be the commonest cause of chronic renal failure.

Urinary tract infection in children is especially worrying. In a study carried out in Charlottesville, Virginia, specimens were collected from about 16,000 different children, about equally divided between the sexes, on one or more occasions. The investigators found bacteria in the urine of 1.2 per cent of the girls and 0.03 per cent of the boys. After treatment, three-quarters of the infections reappeared within two years, while the incidence in girls not infected previously was 0.7 per cent over the same period. It seems that once children have had a urinary tract infection—even one without symptoms—they become more prone to the condition than those who have not been infected before. Moreover, X-rays showed that in 13.7 per cent of 107 of the infected schoolgirls the kidneys had been attacked.

There is thus ample justification for regular mass screening to detect bacteria in the urine, for which simple, reliable techniques already exist. The outlay on a community-wide programme would be substantial. But this must be considered against the mountainous costs of kidney machine centres, which require not only complex equipment and monitoring gear but also a vast back-up of laboratory services and those of transplantation teams. *Prevention and Health* has nothing to say about urinary tract infection.

A condition which merits part of one sentence in *Prevention and Health* is glaucoma, a disease characterised by increased pressure of the fluid inside the eye. It can cause blindness. But the earlier glaucoma is identified and treated, the greater the chance that further deterioration in eyesight can be arrested. Detection is a simple procedure, using an instrument called a tonometer. Why, then, are appropriate nationwide screening programmes not established? Could the reason be that glaucoma rarely occurs at an age when it is likely to have an adverse effect on productivity? Is it simply more economical to maintain blind welfare services for people whose condition remains undetected until it has progressed beyond repair?

Glaucoma is unusual below the age of 40, and reaches its

peak at between 60 and 70. The basic defect is in the drainage mechanism of the eye. This results in rising pressure in the fluid over months or years, gradually but inevitably impairing the blood supply to the optic nerve. By the time a patient approaches his doctor or optician with symptoms the condition is usually far advanced. At that stage, it may continue to worsen despite treatment. But, if detected sufficiently early, the increased pressure inside the eye can be reduced and maintained at its normal level. This prevents further loss of vision. Estimates of the prevalence of glaucoma vary, ranging from 0.02 per cent of the adult population in Japan to 3.1 per cent in the USA. In some countries 27 per cent of blindness is a result of glaucoma, and in Iceland as much as 60 per cent. The only way of cutting these figures is by early diagnosis.

Among other maladies for which screening has been employed are coronary heart disease (changes in the electrocardiograph pattern may indicate incipient disease), lung cancer (which can be detected by X-ray, but is invariably too far advanced for effective treatment by the time it is visible), and cancer of the large bowel and rectum. The latter tumours illustrate one genuine problem about mass screening. These two parts of the body are among the sites most frequently affected by malignancy, and three-quarters of such tumours can be explored directly by the technique of sigmoidoscopy. Thus many of them could probably be identified before symptoms appear if people of the appropriate age—upwards of fifty, when these cancers become more prevalent—were to submit themselves to sigmoidoscopy at intervals. However, the procedure involves the insertion of a tubular sigmoidoscope into the anus and inside the intestine for several inches. 'It is doubtful if the public could ever be persuaded to accept such a programme,' *Prevention and Health* says, 'which is perhaps as well since the resources and expert manpower required are such that population screening by sigmoidoscopy is never likely to be feasible.'

Overall, the potential benefits of mass screening are enormous and unquestioned. Doubts concern the community's

capacity to pay for it. 'At the very worst', writes Professor John
Butterfield, 'screening programmes could find those with the
most significant chronic disease to ensure that they get priority
for treatment . . . At the best, screening programmes will, with
health education, form part of the whole process that must go
forward to attack the ignorance and cope with the disease of
civilisation in our community.' This judgement does, of
course, remind us that screening is likely to be of most value in
coping not with specific pathogens but with maladies associated with our lifestyle.

Is hypertension a disease?

Blood pressure poses a perplexing problem for the advocates of
health screening. 'Secondary hypertension' is a result of
distinct disease, of the kidney perhaps or narrowing of the
aorta (the giant artery through which blood leaves the heart to
pass round the body). But much more common in Western
countries is the condition known as 'essential hypertension'.
This has no apparent specific cause, and doctors dispute continually over whether it should be termed a disease. There is no
normal figure for blood pressure, though life insurance statistics show that the risk of mortality in all age groups rises surely
with each step in the elevation of the readings. Sir George
Pickering has written: 'If we choose to call essential hypertension a disease, it is a disease of a kind hitherto unrecognised by
medicine, a disease characterised by a quantitative, not a
qualitative, deviation from the norm.' Thus a condition that
undoubtedly has adverse effects and shortens lives can in no
way be accounted for by the theory of specific aetiology.
    What we do know about hypertension is that in developed
countries it increases with age. In early life blood pressure in
males tends to be higher than that in females. But from the
age of forty-five onwards women's average blood pressure
becomes higher than that among men. To some extent this
reflects the deaths of hypertensive males; they are much more

likely than women to develop and die of coronary heart disease, fatalities from which are related closely to raised blood pressure. Hypertension is also correlated with obesity. And as we have seen (p. 155), past assumptions that blood pressure rises inevitably with advancing years are by no means valid in communities that have not had the benefits of westernisation.

Should an indistinct condition, one with no particular cause, be treated? Should people with slight or moderate hypertension be identified by screening and converted into patients receiving appropriate drugs? Certainly, the pharmaceutical industry has worked hard to devise drugs for this purpose. The first were introduced in 1949, but the side effects they produced and the need for careful control meant they were unsuitable for all but the most severe cases. More recently, during the late 1950s and early 1960s, two types of drugs have appeared which are considered appropriate for people with blood pressure a little above average but who have no resulting symptoms. The Office of Health Economics, which is financed by the pharmaceutical industry in Britain, is in no doubt that these medicaments should be used widely: 'Attitudes formed when no effective treatment was available may take a long time to adapt to new circumstances. Perhaps the next generation of doctors will be more enthusiastic about the potential benefits from controlling mild or moderate hypertension, especially if further research can isolate specific groups of hypertensives who are particularly at risk.' The late Professor Henry Miller took a different view: 'We do not know whether the rigorous treatment of early asymptomatic hypertension prolongs life or not. What we do know from our experience of insurance examinations is that its detection can cause disabling anxiety.'

There is, in fact, some evidence that drugs have a beneficial effect on marked hypertension without severe symptoms. In the United States, a study under the auspices of the Veterans Administration showed that there were just two serious complications and no deaths among 73 such middle-aged men treated for two and a half years, compared with 27 serious complications and four deaths among 70 men not receiving therapy. Another VA survey demonstrated similar gains from drugs in men with only mild or moderately raised blood pressure without symptoms. The value was mainly in a reduced incidence of strokes. There was no significant fall in the prevalence of coronary heart disease between the treated and untreated groups.

There are good reasons to be cautious about these findings. The men were not a random sample; they were already in contact with the health services and were better motivated than most to accept the undesirable side effects of treatment. 'Unreliable' and 'uncooperative' patients were excluded from the outset. Thus the results may not reflect, either in susceptibility to complications or tolerance of treatment, what one would expect from a random study in the entire population. Other surveys have been equivocal. One British investigation, for example, showed that anti-hypertensive drugs were of no value in a group of middle-aged women. Moreover, statistics based solely on the frequency of severe complications do not take into account the anxiety that can be fostered when an apparently healthy person is turned into an apparently ill patient.

The drug industry is, of course, keen to further the idea that hypertension in any form and of any degree is a disease that should be dealt with by specific therapy. The evidence against this posture is persuasive. And the increasing suspicion that our Western lifestyle alone has turned blood pressure into a problem makes it look particularly bizarre.

Cancer and environment

Doctors have prescribed twenty or so drugs that turned out to be carcinogens. They include chlornaphazine, which causes bladder cancer, anabolic steroids, which can produce liver tumours; and polycyclic hydrocarbons in coal tar ointments, which have caused skin cancer. The majority have been identified quickly, before producing widespread malignancies. One of the most recent and intriguing examples was stilboestrol, which has caused carcinoma of the vagina in young women whose mothers had taken the drug during pregnancy. This association came to light only when a lift broke down in Boston and a gynaecologist and a pathologist met, talked, and pooled their experiences.

Two types of agents used in medicine have resulted in substantial numbers of cancers. Sir Richard Doll calculates that radiation, in the form of X-rays, probably produced between 5 and 10 per cent of all childhood cancers in Western Europe and North America during the 1950s and 1960s, when used for diagnosis during pregnancy. Oestrogens, he also believes, may have done considerable harm. Those given to combat the menopause (see p. 92) may account for much of the recent increase in cancer of the lining of the womb among women in the United States.

Such cases seem extraordinary, because they are examples of iatrogenic disease — that which follows directly from medical treatment. Indeed, they *are* extraordinary. In most instances, the tumours were noted speedily, and the drugs withdrawn, simply because they occurred in people who were already under medical care. But with oestrogen therapy and radiography during pregnancy the dangers took many years to become apparent, because the tumours resembled closely those that result commonly from other causes.

Iatrogenic cancers thus illustrate both the promise and the pitfalls in what is destined to become an increasingly important technique in the fight against malignant disease: the abolition of environmental and dietary hazards. The continued failure of efforts to pinpoint specific causes of cancer, and to fabricate magic bullets to attack tumour tissue, has focused attention on the alternative strategy of eradicating the external agents that are in reality secondary causes. Already, the changed mood is apparent, with authoritative estimates that 80 per cent or more of cancers could be eliminated in this way. But a frustrating difficulty is that there may well be a lengthy time-lag between exposure to a carcinogen and the development of cancer. Decades can elapse before the pattern emerges and evasive measures are adopted.

Most occupational cancers have come to light not from laboratory research but from epidemiological surveys highlighting the clustering of cases. Sometimes, the clusters have been very small and have been noted only as a result of rare perspicacity. Thus Dr John Jones's disquiet at seeing two employees of the Mond Nickel Company develop nasal sinus cancer within a year led to the identification of a hazard from nickel ore. On occasions, however, the risks have been very great. Of one small group of 19 men employed in distilling 2-naphthylamine, 18 died of bladder cancer (the nineteenth was killed in an accident shortly after the disease was diagnosed). This chemical is no longer manufactured. In many other situations, processes have been modified to reduce the occupational hazard. But a debate continues about levels of exposure. A decade ago, the notion of thresholds provided satisfying reassurance. There were specific 'safe levels', below which one could assume complete safety and above which one recognised a danger. Nowadays, we suspect that such a precise guarantee rarely if ever exists. There is a gradation of risk, which grows steadily with increasing exposure. The only truly safe level is no exposure whatever.

Several of the industrial carcinogens also occur in the general environment and so pose a threat not only to factory workers but to all of us. Asbestos, for example, has been found in town air, in particularly high concentration around building sites where it was being sprayed. It is also carried on the clothes of asbestos workers — presumably the source of exposure for the 37 cases of lung cancer that have been detected in household contacts in nine countries. Again, as the hazard — and the absence of a safe threshold — have been appreciated, the authorities have acted to restrict exposure to progressively lower limits. One study of an asbestos textile factory in England showed that the relative danger of lung cancer for men who had been employed for twenty years was ten times normal if they had been employed before 1933 — when the first minor controls became effective. The risk declined to three and a third times normal if they had worked at the factory before 1933 but for less than ten years, and to one and a half times if they had been employed there only after 1933. Yet recent preliminary figures suggest that some risk still persists for men who were first employed only after 1951. Moreover, sawing and drilling asbestos board can pollute the home with asbestos dust, though labelling and precautionary advice are now diminishing this hazard.

Food and drink undoubtedly make their contribution too. Cancer of the mouth attributable to chewing betal and other tasties accounts for a quarter of all cancers in men in parts of India. In the West, the use of preservatives, colouring and sweetening agents has been under suspicion, together with the polycyclic hydrocarbons produced by frying, grilling, and smoking. Sir Richard Doll considers, however, that industrialisation is more likely to have affected cancer incidence via the mass refining of carbohydrates — dietary changes that may be relevant not only to bowel cancer but also to breast cancer, whose geographical pattern remains a puzzle. One explanation of the greater prevalence of breast tumours in Western countries could be that a low residue diet creates conditions in the bowel that encourage bacteria to produce oestrogens.

Vitamins appear to be important in protecting the body against cancer. Two recent studies have shown that deficiency of vitamin A increases the risk of malignancies in the windpipe in smokers. This confirms earlier experiments on animals indicating that the incidence of cancer could be reduced by feeding them a diet enriched in vitamin A, which is supplied richly by foods such as carrots. Fat is also a suspect factor, consumption correlating closely with both colon and breast tumours in different countries. Some evidence suggests that it is linked even more closely with cancer of the lining of the womb. Tumours of the oesophagus, and to a lesser extent the mouth, pharynx and larynx, cause excess mortality among publicans and waiters. Alcohol seems the likely culprit in producing them.

Sir Richard Doll, reviewing such evidence, predicts that the hazards responsible for the majority of human cancers may be detected in future by a combination of epidemiological and laboratory inquiries. Several moves have been made recently in this direction. The World Health Organisation has set up the International Agency for Research on Cancer, and in Britain departments of cancer epidemiology have been established in the universities. 'With this collaboration, a rational use of medical records, and continued support for general biological research,' Sir Richard concludes, 'I see no reason why causes for the remaining common cancers should not be detected within one or two decades. That is not to say that it will be easy to prevent the disease. For if, as I suspect, these hazards are associated with the common diet of developed countries, the problems that we are now having to face in preventing tobacco-induced cancer will seem childishly simple.'

As with cardiovascular disease, it may well be that the real answer has nothing to do with specific causes that can be neutralised by specific antidotes, but is already within our grasp in the form of changes in diet and lifestyle. Which brings us to individual motivation and government persuasion. To what extent should a government interfere with taxation and commercial interests to prevent us from undermining our own health?

Big brother

The Norwegian government has already decided its answer to this question and is experimenting with an integrated nutrition, food and agriculture policy, one aim of which is to reduce the financial and social costs of ill health—especially cardiovascular disease. A particular concern is that deaths from coronary heart disease are increasing among young men, with families to support, who have been trained at public expense and acquired skills that are valuable to the community. The government has decreed that health education is not sufficient to reverse the trend; direct control of pricing will be required if people are to be prevented from consuming too much of the foods that are considered bad for them.

The chief reason why the Norwegians are sceptical of the value of persuasion is that Sweden has failed to effect radical change in this way. Sweden is one of the most intensively screened and doctored countries in the world, with continual scavenging for disease and latent disease in the community. Either because of this, or for genetic reasons, it has one of the best health records of any nation in the world. Compared with Britain, for example, there are considerably fewer infant deaths, and an even greater disparity in mortality rates between the ages of 45 and 64. According to *Prevention and Health*, between a quarter and a third of all of the fatalities in Britain in 1972 would have been avoided if the Swedish mortality rates had applied. Yet coronary heart disease remains a serious problem in Sweden, as in all Western countries, and in 1972 the government launched a 'Diet and Exercise' crusade to persuade its citizens of the value of sensible eating and regular exercising. Several million kroner were spent on the campaign, via schools, newspaper features, television programmes, posters and other means. At first, fat consumption fell—by about 2 per cent. But then it rose again, from 119 grammes per person in 1973 to 124 grammes in 1975. The likely explanation was that while one government department was spending money on health and nutrition education another was providing handsome subsidies to protect Sweden's farmers by increasing people's consumption of beef, butter, cheese, and pork. Taxpayers' money was being used both to discourage citizens from consuming animal fat and to make it easier for them to do so.

Hence the Norwegian government's firmer approach. In its *Report to the Storting No. 32 (1975-76)*, the Royal Norwegian Ministry of Agriculture proposed that consumer education should continue, but be backed by production and pricing policies. One example is action to adjust the nutritional value of both animals and crop plants. About two-thirds of the body fat of intensively reared animals fed on grain is saturated fat, whereas grass-fed animals have only about a third of their fat in the saturated form. Thus, by imposing a levy on imports of feed grains, the government hopes to make farmers use more grass. Consumers should benefit without being conscious of their good fortune. Other government actions may be more obvious and less welcome — like the decision not to subsidise sugar, so that the retail price will reflect the true import price. The plan is for consumption to stabilise at around 70 lb. per year — the 'break point' calculated by Dr Campbell in relation to diabetes (see p. 168), and considerably lower than that in most Western countries today. The loss in energy intake can be compensated for by greater use of cereals.

The Norwegian policy is not a narrow one concerned only with health; it covers questions of housing and population too. Recent years have seen an accelerating migration from the land to the towns; between 1960 and 1973 over 70,000 small farms were abandoned by their owners. The government hopes to slow down and possibly even reverse this trend, thus regaining lost food-producing capacity and curbing the need for new housing and alternative jobs. But its principal aim, as expressed by the Norwegian delegation to the World Food Conference in Rome in November 1974, is to show that 'the diet of the developed countries should not be taken as a model of satisfactory nutrition', and to adopt firm measures accordingly.

Knowledge and action

One of the lessons to be learned from the history of preventive medicine is that even incomplete knowledge may be sufficient to allow effective action. Thus a considerable time elapsed between the discovery of ways of preventing scurvy and cholera and the identification of the specific causes of these conditions. The naval surgeon James Lind found that lime juice forestalled the development of scurvy in 1753 — a century and a half before the isolation and synthesis of vitamin C, the specific active ingredient. John Snow removed the Broad Street pump handle thirty years before Robert Koch identified the cholera bacterium. And in 1775 the surgeon Percivall Pott incriminated coal soot as a cause of cancer of the genital organs in chimney sweeps, but the chemical compound responsible was not identified until the 1930s. Even today, we do not fully understand how chemical carcinogens work.

To a considerable degree, preventive medicine rests not on specialised knowledge of particular causation, but on ideas of hygiene, sanitation, and sensible living that have been appreciated for centuries, together with the simple, well established principles of immunisation. Much of that understanding is not applied. Epidemics of cholera still occur, because water supplies have been contaminated with faeces. Many millions continue to smoke or drink themselves into chronic ill health. High-rise flats are still constructed, despite past experience that habitations of this sort can foster mental disease. Most of us consume a diet that is not only unnatural, in its contrasts with those of our biological predecessors, but also positively harmful. Foolish local authorities continue to resist the fluoridation of water supplies, though we know that this has a striking effect on the quality of our teeth. Venereal disease is flourishing again (penicillin and the magic bullets notwithstanding). Acceptance rates for childhood immunisation against diseases such as poliomyelitis are falling in many countries due to parental apathy. Malaria is thriving and road accidents increasing.

According to the World Health Organisation, one million dollars can educate fifteen doctors. Or it can train 200 auxiliary health workers, largely concerned with preventive medicine. Or it can buy vaccines for a million children. For the countries of the Third World, to which we turn in the next chapter, such choices are very real. The West has been in the comfortable position of being able to afford all three options. But the dominant motif of Western medicine nonetheless has been the specific treatment of identified disorders. Only very recently, stricken by financial stringency, have we seriously begun to investigate major initiatives towards the preventive approach. *Prevention and Health*, indeed, was followed in December 1977 by a UK government White Paper of the same name. It reinforced the arguments in the earlier document that people should be encouraged to take more responsibility for their own health—but went no further than that. Meanwhile, the inappropriateness of the bequest of Western medicine to the Third World is becoming increasingly apparent.

8
Third World medicine

Two personal anecdotes illustrate vividly how incongruous orthodox Western medicine can be when it is transplanted into the Third World. One comes from the late Professor Henry Miller. Even he, a staunch enthusiast for curative high technology, was struck by its irrelevance in a developing country: 'This situation is epitomised by the memory of an evening spent in Bombay when some very elegant electron microscope preparations were demonstrated in a room above a squalidly overcrowded hospital ward and overlooking a street in which people were sleeping huddled in every doorway and on every pavement.'

The other is an incident recorded by Dr Timothy Black after a visit to an aid post in a remote jungle area of New Guinea. One day a woman brought a three-month-old baby boy to Dr Black at the dispensary. The baby, which had a small hernia, was dehydrated and underfed — as was common in an area where mothers were often unable to obtain the protein necessary for a good flow of breast milk. The woman was still suckling an older child, aged about two and a half. Surgery was necessary, but the mother refused adamantly to take her child to the district hospital. She had four young children, she said, and her husband had died recently. She was unable to spend enough time fishing or preparing sago (the local staple diet), while the sale of copra from her few coconut trees did not raise enough money to meet her family's meagre needs. The woman insisted that she could not leave her children and take the baby to hospital. So a compromise was agreed.

Dr Black would carry out the operation at the dispensary.

Everything went well, despite Timothy Black's inexperience, and afterwards he carried the baby out to its mother, who was squatting in the shade of a tree with her other children.

> As I handed her the baby and she saw he was still alive, her face fell in obvious disappointment. My shock was absolute. My immediate reaction was one of utter indignation. The gulf separating my life experience and that of this pitifully poor native woman was complete. She had wanted the baby to die — not to live — during the operation. After my initial outburst, I suddenly realised that I had presented her not only with her baby, but with another mouth to feed — another dependent human being to whom she could offer nothing: no father, no education, no future — merely the cruel ritual of bare survival. It was at that moment I began to realise that preventing a birth could be as important as saving a life.

Water and health

So the specialised expertise of Western medicine can seem insignificant amidst environmental and social problems in the so-called developing world. Other factors have an infinitely greater influence on the pattern of health and ill health. One of the most important is water. Every year, waterborne intestinal diseases cause ten million deaths, and the World Health Organisation estimates that the burden of sickness in the world could be reduced by 80 per cent if everyone had access to potable water. In any community, therapeutic medicine can make no more than marginal contributions to health as long as every drop of water drunk exposes people to further risk of infection. 'Magic bullets' are the most inappropriate missiles imaginable in such a context. What needs to be done is to clean up the water supply, not attack particular pathogenic targets one by one.

Schistosomiasis, the most widespread of parasitic afflictions, is a waterborne condition for which conventional curative medicine may never provide an answer. It is pre-eminently an environmental disease, affecting 200 million people in 71 countries. The cause is a minute flat worm which spends part of its life cycle in man and part in the water snail. Infected individuals excrete the eggs of the parasite. In insanitary conditions, these find their way into water, where they hatch into 'miracidia' which then invade the water snail. After further developmental stages, forked tailed 'cercariae' appear. When they encounter feet or other human tissues, these digest their way through the skin, into the bloodstream, and through the heart to the lungs. They may live inside the blood vessels of various internal organs for many years, releasing eggs through both urine and faeces — initiating further cycles of infection. The disease is a debilitating malady, destroying energy and initiative rather than killing its victims. It can be treated, though complete cure is a rarity. Chemicals may be used to destroy the snails in watercourses. But this is relatively inefficient, it is costly, and the environmental consequences are unpredictable. The surer answer is to prevent human waste from reaching water with which people have contact. The snail's habitat can also be tackled, by draining irrigation channels, by cutting bankside vegetation to ensure a rapid flow of water, and by changing the course of watercourses (see p. 203). Control of schistosomiasis is thus inextricably bound up with sanitation, land and water management, and agriculture. It has nothing to do with specific aetiology.

Self-help in Sarawak

Such environmental health hazards are often tackled most effectively by self-help. One example is the remarkable results achieved in recent years in Sarawak under the Rural Health Improvement Scheme, helped by WHO and UNICEF. Until 1967 sanitary facilities simply did not exist in the country's villages. People defecated in the bushes near their homes or directly from their houses on to the ground. Scavenger animals did the work of disposal. Human and animal excreta and refuse fouled the compounds, while water was drawn from nearby polluted streams. Parasitic worms infected 90 per cent of the rural population. Water- and food-borne diseases such as typhoid fever and dysentery were rife.

The key to the conspicuous improvements since that time has been the provision of water supplies as an incentive to persuade people to help themselves. Water taps have been fixed in individual kitchens in the kampongs (longhouses)— but only when the occupants have asked for a supply and have undertaken to contribute money and free labour to build and maintain the system, to construct sanitary toilets, and to dig drainage ditches and fence in their pigs. One village, Kampong Skiat, with a population of 200, had always obtained its water from the bottom of the hill. Then in 1974 the people raised money and asked the government to install piped water. Staff from the Rural Health Improvement Scheme surveyed the area and found a spring about a mile away. The villagers themselves helped to construct the pipeline. Today every dwelling in the kampong has fresh water and a sanitary toilet—and the women have been spared the back-breaking task of carrying water up the hill each day. Already 1,000 or so water systems have been constructed and by 1980 at least half of the 750,000 people in Sarawak's 2,800 kampongs should have water taps and proper lavatories.

Efforts to improve rural health actually began in Sarawak in the early 1960s, but people responded poorly at first. At that stage health education was used to promote personal hygiene. Only when clean water was offered as the incentive did folk become really interested. 'Motivators' have been important too, in the form of young men trained to boost the programme by harnessing people's energy and enthusiasm. Trainees with at least nine years of elementary schooling are given a nine-month course on environmental sanitation, mainly on the principles and techniques of water supply, refuse disposal and latrine construction. After training, they return to their own villages and help with tuberculosis and malaria control, care of mothers and children, and first aid, as well as directing water and sanitation projects. Every year they attend a refresher course. They are not imported specialists. They know better than visiting experts can ever know the people, their problems, customs and traditions.

Appropriate sanitation

Provision of clean water is one Western contribution to the Third World whose value is not in dispute. Waterborne disposal of excreta is more contentious. WHO statistics show that only 28 per cent of the urban population of developing countries are served by waterborne sewerage, and that 29 per cent have no sanitation whatever. But flush toilets—which the WHO assumes are both feasible and appropriate for all peoples throughout the world—are extremely wasteful. They consume up to 20 litres per flush, and account for 40 per cent of residential water use where they are employed widely. Moreover, effective alternatives exist. These include composting toilets, which produce clean, rich fertiliser, and various types of fermentation tanks generating methane gas as well as fertiliser. There are also incinerating lavatories that leave only a fine ash, as well as oil-flushing toilets whose oil recycles continuously.

One UK expert who challenges the WHO's strategy of encouraging waterborne sewerage universally is Dr Richard Feacham, of the University of Birmingham. He points out that most developing countries already find it impossible to create new waterborne facilities at a rate that keeps pace with their urban population growth, let alone provide them for existing slum dwellers. Cost is a major drawback. Most high-density, low-income communities have been unable or unwilling to cover the real capital and running costs of waterborne sewerage in their rates, and city and town authorities are reluctant to subsidise urban sanitation for the poor. The extravagent use of water may be tolerable in a country with ample resources. It is less justifiable in many developing countries, where water is scarce and expensive. There are, in addition, problems such as blockage and those of house demolition when sewers are being layed.

All of these arguments, reminiscent of the views of Mahatma Gandhi, point in the direction of on-site methods for disposing of sewage or for exploiting it as a resource. The communal aqua privy connected to a soak-away, for example, has been tried in several countries, particularly Botswana and Zambia. As yet, such systems are far from ideal, but Dr Feacham argues that development work could well make the aqua privy both acceptable and inexpensive. The need for research in this area is abundantly obvious. Between now and the end of the century, some way must be found to dispose of the human waste of 2.5 million urban dwellers in the developing countries alone. That figure includes people who at present have neither sewage connections nor household systems, those expected to migrate to the cities during the next two decades, and predicted population increases. Neither our financial nor our hydrological resources will be able to cope with this burden by using the most expensive and wasteful sewerage system that now exists.

Simple medicine in Solo

The political and financial priorities, it seems, are very different when we are considering medicine in the Third World from those that have come to dominate Western medicine over the past century. Three case studies will make this clear. First, there is the experience of Dr Gunawan Nugroho working in the government service in Indonesia. Dr Nugroho was appointed in 1963 to the Foundation for Christian Hospitals in Solo, the second largest city in central Java, with a population of about 400,000. At that time the foundation had a small maternity clinic and outpatient clinic attached, on the outskirts of the city, attended by patients from the city and the surrounding villages.

Dr Nugroho soon decided that 'the problem of health was not exclusively one of disease alone; health had a very close relationship with all aspects of life, and a health programme should promote the concept of how to live healthily'. His aim was to focus less on the individual than on the community as a whole, and to make the provision of health services less dependent on overseas experts and aid. And, though the maternity clinic was upgraded into a hospital, expensive and complex equipment was avoided. In place of an incubator, for example, a glass box heated with an electric lamp was used, because most of the auxiliary staff were untrained village girls. One major snag that came to light early on was that the under-privileged members of the community were excluded from the health service provided at the hospital, mainly by its cost. Because meetings arranged to discuss this with community leaders were 'misinterpreted politically', the first efforts to create a community health programme with greater participation failed. Dr Nugroho resolved that he must spend more time in the field, while his wife ran the hospital.

Begajah, a village of about 3,500 inhabitants twenty kilometres south of Solo, typified the problems. Many adult patients came from there to the outpatients clinics with various forms of malnutrition. The infant mortality rate was around 100 per 1,000 and a sizeable proportion of children suffered from malnutrition too. The glaringly obvious problem was not a want of specific therapies but a dire shortage of food. In 1966 the average family holding was 0.2 hectares of irrigated rice land and 0.1 hectares of dry land. This could produce enough for the family to subsist on — 480 kilograms of rice and 175 kilos of soy bean, peanut, sweet potatoes, corn and other products — if the weather was favourable. Heavy rains or a long drought could be disastrous. So a village development committee was established. Using new rice strains, fertilisers and appropriate agricultural methods on a demonstration plot, the committee showed how yields could be boosted greatly. And through a 'food for work' programme, whereby the community provided labour in return for Bulgar wheat, the irrigation system was improved. Rice production doubled, from 442 tons in 1966 to 854 tons in 1970. Infant mortality fell to 69 per 1,000, and a survey during 1970 revealed not a single case of malnutrition. Increased agricultural productivity, backed by health and nutrition education, had transformed the health of the community.

Moreover, such measures were highly cost-effective. In 1969, for example, the community received 9.8 tons of Bulgar wheat for work in improving irrigation canals. This increased the average yield by 31 per cent. Dr Nugroho concluded: 'For the first time it has been proved that a comprehensive approach in raising health standards through community development with community participation could be implemented, and was cheap and appropriate.' Following this and similar successes, Indonesia has also been introducing community-based health insurance, centred on the idea of prepaid medical care. Monthly contributions are very small, but these payments are only one part of the schemes, which depend for their success on the promotion of awareness and a sense of responsibility. 'A community health programme directs its attention to health rather than disease and focuses not only on the individual but rather on the community,' Dr Nugroho insists. 'The well-being of the community can be more quickly attained if all its members unite their efforts so as to create conditions whereby the community can progress towards greater welfare.

Revolution in Mozambique

Another country that has seen radical efforts to change the balance of its health care is Mozambique. Following ten years of guerilla warfare against the Portuguese, colonial rule ended towards the end of September 1974. One immediate result was the near collapse of all medical services as many white doctors and scientists left the country. Since then the new government has made concerted attempts to swing the emphasis from curative medicine towards the prevention of disease.

The starting-point was a medical 'service' which had left 70 per cent of the people without doctors, hospitals, or even rudimentary health care. But during the decade of fighting the FRELIMO leaders had come to know at first hand the lives of the people in the rural areas, their malnutrition, ignorance and endemic disease. The inequality between town and country was appalling. On the one hand there were hospitals with sophisticated equipment in Maputo, Beira, and Nampula, providing medical care for the privileged few; on the other, a lack of the most basic facilities. The medical services that did obtain were entirely curative; disease prevention was non-existent. And this despite the fact that the infections that dominate the pattern of ill health in Mozambique are those for which preventive measures can win rich rewards very quickly. Mass vaccination programmes and projects designed to raise standards of hygiene and change people's living conditions have been corner-stones of the new government's health policy. Auxiliaries, rather than doctors, are the key workers in carrying through the preventive work. The major achievement to date has been a vaccination campaign, funded by UNICEF, the aim of which is to immunise the entire population against measles, tuberculosis and smallpox.

But, as in Solo, medicine *per se* is not first on the list of national priorities. The government has placed agriculture first, education second, and health third. In the long term, however, the greatest progress in the third area will come via advances in the other two. The Minister of Health, Dr Helder Martins, explains:

Health is a political problem, particularly where preventive medicine is concerned. Health structures are reflections of society, so political structures are our best instruments to develop a programme of health care. If the Ministry of

Health had embarked on health education as a purely technical operation, it could never have got through to the mass of the population. The most difficult thing is to change people's mentalities. In switching from curative to preventive medicine, the most difficult obstacle was the health personnel. They had been trained in curative medicine. To persuade them it is cheaper, more humane to prevent than to cure disease, that's difficult.

One part of the plan is for Mozambique's hospitals to switch their role, to act less as preserves of sophisticated medical science and more as bases from which doctors, nurses and auxiliaries can go out into the community to preach health and hygiene. The community, in return, will strengthen this link by providing volunteers to help in cleaning and other work. Another development is the training of large numbers of 'community health promoters', recruited from villagers who can read and write. After four or six months' training in basic hygiene, health and preventive medicine, they will go back to their home villages to advise on everything from farming techniques to malaria prevention. They will require only simple equipment and no base. But they will know the people well, living and working in the community, and the hope is that they will be more successful than outsiders in mobilising health and hygiene efforts in the community.

A few days travelling on the pitted dirt tracks used as roads in provincial Mozambique persuaded one recent visitor, Dr Geoff Watts, that 'civil engineering is as central to the development of rural health as hypodermics and bandages'. Quite simply, transport problems are among the greatest obstacles to the development of rural health services in the country. As an example of the difficulties Dr Watts instanced, plans to build a new *infantario* (a cross between an orphanage and a kindergarten) in the Niassa province in northern Mozambique. The existing *infantario*, in which over a hundred children lived, consisted of two long decrepit tin shacks, without a proper kitchen or laundry. Half a mile away the government had laid out the ground for a new building which should have taken eighteen months to complete. But every bag of cement, every door knob and every other item needed for construction had to be brought more than 300 kilometres over roads impassable in wet weather and punishingly bad in the dry season. The country is also chronically short of both building materials and skilled men.

Transport, building materials, food supply and sewage disposal have nothing to do with specific aetiology. But in developing countries they are of incomparably greater significance for the health of the people.

A Latin-American view

A third impression of medicine in the Third World was recorded by Paul Harrison, on the basis of visits to two basic health projects in Latin America during 1976. One was the MAC (Module for Amplification of Coverage) system in Colombia, which he observed in a hillside slum settlement overlooking the capital, Bogota. The other, around Lake Titicaca, was part of an Integrated Services Project run jointly by UNICEF and the Peruvian government. Both were set up for the same reason — the health of the rural peoples was mediocre and was seen increasingly as a barrier to economic development. As in our other two examples, principal underlying causes of death and disease were malnutrition and poor sanitation. From a Western perspective, particular gastrointestinal and respiratory pathogens were to blame. But there is little point in deploying specific therapies against such agents in a community where unhygienic conditions ensure continual reinfection, and where at the same time scarcity of food erodes people's resistance.

Both Latin-American programmes emphasise prevention, via nutrition and sanitation. Both focus primarily on the poor rural population and on mothers and children. And both rely heavily on 'health promoters' who (as laid down in UNICEF/

WHO guidelines issued in 1975) require at least seven years' schooling and are trusted local residents. In Colombia they must have lived for five years in the area they serve and in Peru they are elected by the community. Their duties include sanitation and nutrition education, based on self-help in the community, as well as immunisations, first aid, and midwifery.

The *Health Promoter's Manual* used in Peru illustrates the basic level of the teaching:

> A man with diarrhoea goes to the riverside. A pig eats his faeces and tramples it with its feet. Then the pig goes into a house. A child is playing on the floor where the pig is walking—so the child dirties itself with the crap of the sick man. The child cries, so his mother picks him up. Then she peels potatoes, forgetting to wash her hands. All the family eats the potatoes. Then all the family catches diarrhoea.

Not a word here about *Salmonella typhimurium*. No need for it. No need, either, for the specialised laboratory technology that allows individual substrains of *S. typhimurium* to be identified with discrimination and precision. Gastro-intestinal disease can be combated very effectively without all that. The special knowledge the manual *does* impart is how to rehydrate and feed children with diarrhoea—again, non-specific skills, but vitally important ones (see p. 208).

As Harrison found, however, the injunctions of preventive medicine are not always heeded in a society where people accept known health risks as an inevitable part of life. Thus many slum dwellers in Bogota consciously choose to live in an area lacking a clean water supply because rents in districts with piped water are too high.

> They are willing to trade off the certainty of a present saving against the mere possibility of future disease ... Prevention and even cure are not self evident necessities—everything hinges on their cost, relative to the cost of suffering illness.

It may, in fact, be cheapest of all to accept illness, next cheapest to seek a traditional cure, relatively dear to seek even a basic health care cure, and dearest of all to take preventive action.

Health promoters could transform this situation, ensuring that families which do not consult doctors at present will begin to make some use of the health services. This will be particularly important for children. Whereas illness in an adult can mean loss of earnings, in a child it may bring economic benefits — one mouth less to feed. But in Colombia and Peru, as throughout the Third World, preventive medicine furthered by health promoters is unlikely to be anywhere near fully effective unless it is accompanied by two other initiatives: the energetic promotion of family planning and the provision of health insurance and financial aid to help people apply preventive principles. Even the simple act of boiling water for a baby's bottle costs money.

The Chinese experience

The country that has gone furthest to renounce specialisation in medicine, and foster the preventive approach 'in the field', is the People's Republic of China. In 1949, the health of the Chinese people — 80 per cent of them living in rural areas — was desperately poor. The civil conflict and years of war with Japan had exacerbated disease problems arising from infectious disease and poverty. Up to 200 out of every 1,000 infants died in the first year of life, and an estimated 30 per cent of children did not survive to the age of five. The new communist government decided that to tackle such problems by expanding conventional medical resources would have been a never-ending, perhaps impossible, task. It also recognised the importance of health services for production. So the strategy adopted was that of mobilising the people themselves towards preventive measures. The four guiding principles laid down by the First and Second National Health Conferences in 1950 and 1951 were: 'serve the workers, peasants, and soldiers'; 'place the chief emphasis on prevention'; 'stress co-operation between doctors of Western and traditional medicine'; and 'rely on mass movements for the carrying out of health work'.

A key role is played by 'barefoot doctors'—so named because in the south the peasants work in barefoot in the rice paddies. Barefoot doctors are peasants who receive a basic medical training, and they carry out their duties without leaving productive work. In this they differ from medical auxiliaries like the feldshers in Russia, who form a group separate from their patients. Barefoot doctors spend at least half of their time doing agricultural work—much more at harvest and planting time. Their pay is the same as that of their non-medical fellows, which in turn depends on the income of the commune.

Barefoot doctors are responsible for environmental sanitation, health education, immunisation, first aid, and some aspects of basic medical care for ill people. They have to supervise the proper collection, treatment, storage and use of human faeces as fertiliser. They direct campaigns against disease vectors such as snails and flies and are skilled in diagnosing and treating minor and common illnesses. During their six months' training they are shown how infectious diseases spread and take basic courses in anatomy and physiology. They become acquainted with traditional herbal remedies as well as antibiotics, with syringes as well as acupuncture needles.

A major landmark in Chinese medical care came in 1965 with Chairman Mao's 'June 26 Directive' in which he instructed that 'the central gravity of health work be shifted to the countryside'. Barefoot doctors had existed previously but after that time they became central to Chinese medicine. The rationale is indisputable. Faced with the choice, it is better to establish mass care that is competent to deal with 90 per cent of disease (though resulting in a small percentage of errors) than to provide specialised medical attention for only a tiny percentage of the population. Moreover, as Dr Peter Wilenski points out, 'any debate over quality versus quantity in rural medical care has to take into account the questionable effectiveness of the academically trained doctor because of his difficulties in communication and lack of awareness of the patients' social conditions'. This status and language gap can be potent in thwarting the translation of medical knowledge into action. Even in the United States, better health results have been obtained in Mexican-American communities by employing agricultural workers after a short period of training as health leaders than by using 'professionals'.

Community action is another plank of Chinese medical care. Efforts to eradicate schistosomiasis are typical. In 1955, over 10.4 million people in Shanghai and twelve provinces along the mouth of the Yangtze River were infested with the disease. In some villages 70 per cent of the population were infected. So the government decreed that the masses should be mobilised to fight the pestilence. Large numbers of workers, not specific chemical poisons, were the weapons. There was opposition to the idea at first. The government denounced this later as the 'bourgeois reactionary line ... which ... relies on a small number of "specialists" and professionals working in isolation from the masses'. But the scheme went ahead, and chemicals such as sodium pentachlorophenate and calcium cyanide, lethal to the snails which carry the parasites, were not used. The most dramatic results came from efforts to change the snails' environment so that they could not survive. As they cannot re-emerge from under a layer of 10 cm of earth, the commonest method was to bury them. Peasants went into the fields and lowered the water level in streams and irrigation ditches by blocking the flow temporarily. They dug ditches along the sides, dumping the surface earth at the bottom of the channel, and then buried this with fresh earth. In one campaign in Anhwei province in 1956, 1½ million people were reported to have devoted 20 million man-days to the work.

Another stratagem was to destroy the parasites' eggs in human faeces—which in China are valued as a fertiliser to be

204 Beyond the magic bullet

used in rice fields. Faeces were formerly stored in pots or jars (which often overflowed) along river banks or near rice fields. This was one way in which the eggs were spread. Then some- one found that a mixture of faeces and urine, kept for a few days, generates ammonia, which destroys the eggs. So new methods of storage were introduced. Individual families were made responsible for controlling strictly the disposal of their faeces — propaganda *and* cash incentives being employed to make sure that the job was done properly. In some areas, local control centres bought and collected the 'night soil', retained it for a period until the eggs were dead, and then let the peasants use it as fertiliser. Other measures included the building of public latrines (over 60 million in the first nine months of 1958) and the penning of animals in separate enclosures.

The Chinese authorities report that by the end of 1959 work to eradicate snails had been extended successfully over a region of 6,350 million square metres. Many areas had been declared free. Since then progress seems not to have been maintained, because the Cultural Revolution of 1966-8 disrupted anti- schistosomiasis work. The disease then reappeared in some areas where it had been brought under control. In an indepen- dent assessment in 1976 Dr Wilenski concluded that 'there can be little doubt that even if the Chinese claims of imminent eradication of the disease have been premature, inexpensive labour-intensive methods have resulted in a major improve- ment in health in the 12 affected provinces.'

What the Chinese seem to have done in their schistosomiasis and other crusades is to mobilise previously untapped labour in the countryside. As in many developing countries, the marginal productivity of this labour force was low, but by their patriotic campaigns the Chinese leaders have managed to exploit this 'surplus' labour for work towards the greater health of the community. Together with moves to end the compart- mentalisation of medical knowledge, they have created a sense of individual and community responsibility for health. Infant mortality rates have fallen and eradication programmes against diseases such as malaria and kala-azar (a disease similar to malaria, transmitted by sand flies) have proved successful. Many visitors report that sanitary conditions in both the cities and countryside have been transformed over the past two or three decades. Dr Wilenski concludes: 'The patriotic health movement has been based on a unique combination of epidemiological knowledge and sociopolitical action to achieve considerable results in community health with a minimum of scarce resources.'

Medicines and the market

The inappropriateness in the Third World of much Western medicine, founded on the rock of specific aetiology, is exemplified by some of the activities of Western-based multinational pharmaceutical companies in developing countries. Here commerce promotes the deployment of magic bullets at the expense of attention to the real environmental and social determinants of ill health. It often does so with callous disregard for the consequences. One of the most horrifying aspects of the thalidomide affair in the late 1950s and early 1960s was the different standards of conduct adopted by one of the manufacturers, the Astra Company, in Scandinavia and in its export market in Argentina. The promotional literature distributed to doctors in Sweden, Denmark, and Norway was moderate in tone, avoiding far-reaching claims about the safety of the tranquilliser thalidomide. Corresponding material used in Argentina was unrestrained. And, although the Astra Company withdrew the drug at home in Scandinavia at the beginning of December 1961, it did not reach a similar decision regarding sales in Argentina until March 1962.

One man who has made a special study of the conduct of drug houses in different parts of the globe is Dr Milton Silverman. A journalist as well as a pharmacologist, he has worked for the US Public Health Service, and his book *The Drugging of the Americas*, published in 1976 is a systematic comparison of drug literature in the USA and in Latin

America. It is a frightening document. Dr Silverman contrasted the promotional material for twenty-eight important,
widely used drugs in the USA and in Brazil, Mexico, and other
Latin-American countries. He used as his sources the
Physician's Desk Reference (the US doctors' 'bible') and comparable volumes, particularly the *Para Los Médicos*, for Latin
America. These contain information provided by drug companies about indications — the symptoms and signs calling for
use of a drug; contra-indications — grounds for *not* administering it; and side-effects — unwelcome and often dangerous
complications, ranging from skin rashes to serious blood
disorders. Again and again, he found the indications listed for
drug prescribing in Latin America were far more extensive
than those issued by the same companies in the United States.
Hazards were correspondingly played down or omitted
altogether. In some instances, trivial side-effects rated a mention, while serious or possibly fatal reactions were not
described.

The antimicrobial drug chloramphenicol is one example.
The *PDR* used large type to warn readers that it should be
used only in serious or life-threatening infections when less
potentially dangerous drugs were ineffective or contraindicated. The risk of aplastic anaemia and other blood diseases was emphasised. Latin American doctors, however, were
told that Parke-Davis's chloramphenicol was indicated not
only for acute typhoid fever but also for abscesses, tonsilitis,
pharyngitis, and many other common infections. Contraindications and adverse reactions were minimised. Some of the
Latin-American descriptions listed a few adverse reactions; in
certain cases none at all were given.

There could be no more graphic illustration of inappropriate medication. As we have seen (p. 75), chloramphenicol
is a valuable drug, which should be reserved for the treatment
of typhoid fever. Yet in the Third World it is being recommended and used to treat other specific conditions — in particular
less serious gastro-intestinal infections that should be prevented in the first place by good hygiene and sanitation. The ill

consequences are twofold: avoidable blood disorders and the proliferation of bacteria resistant to the drug.

Ciba-Geigy's Butazolidin was another of Dr Silverman's examples. In the USA it was recommended for certain severe arthritic conditions. Doctors were told not to use it as a simple analgesic; they were warned of its hazards and advised that treatment should generally be limited to a brief period, particularly in the elderly. Yet possibilities of adverse reactions were not mentioned in some Latin American countries, where the indications for use were much wider. Chlorpromazine, too, was listed in the USA for a restricted list of conditions such as manic-depressive illness. But doctors in the Argentine were advised to use it for hypertension, 'anguish', and 'essential and symptomatic painful conditions'. Compared with the fourteen contra-indications and warnings listed in the USA, the Argentine literature mentioned only comatose states and the presence of large quantities of chemicals depressing the central nervous system. In Brazil the manual did not even mention this danger. The sole warning there appeared to be that during the initial days of treatment with the injectable form of chlorpromazine, especially in those with high or low blood pressure, patients should remain horizontal for half an hour after receiving the dose.

The routine reply by pharmaceutical manufacturers to criticism of this nature is that they abide by the law—that they stick scrupulously to the labelling standards insisted upon by regulatory agencies in whatever country they operate. There are two replies to that plea. First, as Dr Silverman has shown, in some cases drug firms do indeed violate laws requiring hazards to be disclosed. Second, even in countries without such laws—and in those where laws exist but the authorities have chosen not to apply them—pharmaceutical companies have a clear moral obligation to adopt rules of behaviour just as rigorous as those they adopt in Europe and the USA.

Dehydration and rehydration

An outstanding example of a specific remedy that is promoted
and used in a Third World context where it is not a remedy at
all is Lomotil. Produced by a US-based multinational, G. D.
Searle, Lomotil is an anti-diarrhoeal drug which works by
paralysing the gut for several hours and stopping excretion. It
can be invaluable for the travelling executive who is stricken by
the runs on arrival in Delhi with two days of important business meetings to get through. What Lomotil does not do is to
cure gastro-intestinal infections acquired through filthy food
or water. It is an apparently specific remedy for a *condition*,
diarrhoea, but is no answer to the acute diarrhoeal *diseases*
that loom large as causes of death in many Third World countries. There, the appropriate answers are sanitary measures to
prevent the continual transmission of bacteria and other
enteric organisms, and rehydration to replenish fluids in the
unfortunate victims. Yet Lomotil is being promoted energeti-
cally throughout the Third World. Chemists' shops in
Khartoum, for example, carry over-the-counter packs with the
words: 'Lomotil stops diarrhoea fast — as used by astronauts
during Gemini and Apollo space flights.'

Moreover, Lomotil can be dangerous in children. Professor
Colin Forbes, of Nairobi University's Medical Faculty, reports:

> I have seen children poisoned by Lomotil, and there are
> many documented cases. The use of Lomotil in a child is
> bad (and dangerous) medicine. It paralyses the gut and so
> pools the noxious secretions in an inert 'third space', when
> all this fluid is best shat out of the body. Diarrhoea doesn't
> kill children, dehydration does, and Lomotil does not stop
> dehydration. It can allow the child to die of respiratory
> depression and dehydration.

The Lancet has warned: 'The management of acute diarrhoea
in children is essentially dietary, with adequate fluid and
electrolyte salt intake keeping pace with fluid loss. Unnecessary

drug prescription for these children should be vigorously opposed.'

The real answer to much of the childhood diarrhoea of the Third World is not quasi-specific drug therapy, but simple general measures to replenish fluid. When the body loses water and salt through diarrhoea to the extent of 10 per cent of its weight, dehydration becomes severe. Without treatment the victim will then die within an hour or two. What the body needs is water, together with two salts (sodium and potassium chloride) and glucose. Despite the diarrhoea, the gut can still absorb these substances. In severe cases, fluids may have to be replaced by injecting them, like a blood transfusion. Usually, drinking water with a pinch of salt and some orange juice will suffice. A considerable amount of research is now in progress into the best methods of rehydration but the benefits are already clear. Dr S. Suharjono, at Jakarta General Hospital, reports that cholera mortality has fallen from 4 per cent to zero thanks to rehydration — among those victims fortunate enough to be admitted to hospital. The Indonesian approach termed ROSE (Rehydration, including Oral Sustenance, and Education) is partly preventive. People are urged to take a simple, home-made mixture when diarrhoea first begins.

The efficacy of rehydration was demonstrated vividly during the desperate situation that developed in India in 1971, when refugees suffering from cholera and other severe diarrhoeal diseases entered the country from its eastern border. Health services were already severely strained, and this additional load threatened to stretch them to breaking-point. Until that time, the routine approach had always been to replace fluids by injection, but this was out of the question in the refugee camps. There was nothing like sufficient sterile intravenous fluid. Nor were trained staff available to administer it. So the health officer in charge of one camp decided to change over to rehydration by mouth, reserving intravenous fluids for severely dehydrated victims who were in a state of shock. The decision was amply vindicated. Nearly 4,000 patients were brought to the centre over a period of eight weeks, two-fifths of them under the age of five. Of these 135 died (half of them before treatment could begin) — a fatality rate of 3 per cent. The rate for the refugee population as a whole was 30 per cent.

The new technique was developed at the Calcutta Infectious Diseases Hospital and the Dacca Cholera Research Laboratories. It has now become official WHO policy to recommend the use of a simple rehydration solution consisting of sodium and potassium chloride, sodium bicarbonate (baking soda) and glucose — dissolved in clean water. UNICEF has launched a programme to make this formulation available in aluminium packages under the name 'Oralyte' and to promote its local production. A WHO guide on the management of dehydration is being distributed widely as part of its scheme to disseminate simple and effective health techniques to be adapted by different countries and used in extending primary medical care to previously neglected rural and urban communities.

Do we need drugs?

In 1976 the Haslemere Group, in conjunction with War on Want and Third World First, published the report *Who Needs the Drug Companies?* which focused further light on the futility of much of the specific-curative medicine practised in developing countries. A typical case cited is that of the man with hookworm anaemia, who becomes disabled progressively by his illness over the years until he is forced to give up work completely. Admitted to hospital, he requires sophisticated laboratory tests, skilled medical and nursing attention and treatment with drugs. In time he becomes well enough to go back to work again. But the man's living conditions are as bad as they were before and he catches hookworm again. The medical attention he has received — at considerable expense to a struggling Third World economy — has had little real effect. Yet he would probably not have contracted hookworm in the first place if his village had used pit latrines.

The lassitude produced by such chronic, recurring diseases as hookworm anaemia, schistosomiasis and malaria has a massive effect on the economic and social life of Third World countries. These are also the infections that respond dramatically to environmental improvements and preventive measures. The Haslemere Group summarises its indictment as follows:

We have exported to Third World countries, along with the rest of Western medical practice, our own mistaken belief in the efficacy of chemical intervention for individual sufferers from endemic diseases. Third World countries continue to deploy large amounts of their scarce resources on buying drugs from Western countries, often at higher absolute cost than agencies in industrialised countries. Where health and social welfare budgets are low, the high cost of medicines puts them well out of reach of much of the population. Where governments pay for drugs, the cost takes up a disproportionately high amount of the total money available for health, to the detriment of preventive medicine schemes.

The United Nations has estimated that about a quarter of the population of the Western hemisphere lives in countries where the average number of calories and the weight of protein available to each individual is below the levels needed for health. But the corresponding figures for Africa and Asia are 80 and 90 per cent. And there is no specific therapeutic cure for malnutrition. Only social and economic moves will change the diets of the masses of the world's peoples. The Haslemere group declares that the two most important of such moves are alterations in the pattern of land tenure — to favour food production for local populations rather than cash crops for export — and higher investment in the agricultural sector — to increase productivity. 'These are of course questions of social as opposed to medical policy, yet ultimately it is these issues that will most crucially determine the health prospects of underdeveloped countries.'

The Haslemere Group report does not prove that drugs and

drug companies are unnecessary. It does suggest that at most they can make only a marginal impact on health in the Third World. The major causes of death in Third World countries are not obscure tropical diseases. They are acute infections once common in the West, such as measles and tuberculosis, turned into widespread killers by malnutrition and poverty. True, there are tropical infections, for which drug companies like Hoffman La Roche are doing valuable work in developing specific therapies. Thus Roche introduced Astiban in 1961 to treat schistosomiasis, followed shortly afterwards by Fansidar, an antimalarial drug devised as an answer to the resistance of the malarial parasite to the earlier drug, chloroquine. But such infections can be dealt with very much more effectively by environmental and preventive action.

The importance of social factors in the Third World is exemplified by one of the best known and most ancient of tropical infections: leprosy. Effective drugs *are* available yet in India alone some 3.2 million people are still infected with the disease. Findings reported in 1976 from a study in the Chingleput district of Tamil Nadu state, South India, showed that at least half of known leprosy patients do not attend their leprosy centres to receive their monthly supply of dapsone tablets. Interviews with 120 of these patients revealed that their main reason for not attending was a belief in the possibility of self-cure; the disease may regress in the early stages, when the main symptom is numbness, giving the appearance of improvement. Equally important was the nuisance of having to travel — perhaps for a whole day, involving loss of earnings — to a specialist centre. A third reason was that dapsone causes burning stomach pains in many patients — but usually only in those restricted to a single meal each day.

The drug companies *are* needed. So too is specialised expertise throughout the field of health care, from detailed understanding of malnutrition to improvements in techniques of fluid replacement for victims of diarrhoeal disease. But at present many specific remedies, and agents masquerading as such, are being peddled by the pharmaceutical multinationals in the Third World to the long-term detriment of the people's health. And a beguiling belief in the efficacy of specific drug therapy is diverting both money and attention away from the measures that can be dramatically successful in promoting health in the Third World.

Malnutrition and the brain

Only very recently have we become aware of the far-reaching effects of malnutrition in children, not only in impairing the body's defences against infection but also in damaging the developing brain. Until a decade or so ago biologists believed that the growth and basic organisation of the brain took place almost entirely before birth — and that even the brain of a baby inside the womb of an ill-fed mother was protected naturally against harm. Now, due largely to studies by Professor John Dobbing and others at the University of Manchester, we know that at least 80 per cent of human brain development occurs in the first two years of life. During that period malnutrition can damage the brain permanently, impairing intellect later on.

Dobbing's discovery has helped to clarify previously uncertain, anecdotal reports that poorly nourished children are often mentally backward when they grow up. Such findings have been difficult to interpret because of other adverse environmental and social factors that could have been responsible. Two surveys have now confirmed the anecdotes and supported John Dobbing's conclusions. One began in 1966 in a Mexican village of 5,500 people. Joaquín Cravioto, professor of paediatrics at the University of Mexico, was in charge. He selected the 300 children born during a single year in the village — chosen as a place where malnutrition was common. Over seven years, Professor Cravioto and his colleagues recorded the weight, height and health of the infants as well as details of their families. As a measure of the infants' intellectual progress he used a test devised by the American psychologist Francis Palmer which explores the development of

conceptual thought by testing children for their knowledge of
opposites — wet/dry, black/white and so on.

During the first five years of the project, 15 of the children
showed signs of kwashiorkor — a protein deficiency condition in
which the belly protrudes, the limbs swell and the skin cracks.
Another 7 began suffering from the other form of malnutrition, marasmus, characterised by wasting of the muscles.
Given medical care, 19 of the 22 survived. The effects of these
bodily insults on the children's minds seemed unambiguous.
At the age of three, the infants who had experienced kwashiorkor or marasmus had an average language development
score of 657 — compared with 947 for a matched group who
had not apparently suffered malnutrition. There was a 'lag' in
the children's intellectual progress which persisted even after
their physical condition was considered cured.

A second project, carried out by Professor Jack Tizard and
his colleagues with a group of Jamaican infants, gave similar
results. It also confirmed that there is an interplay between
undernutrition and lack of a stimulating environment con-
ducive to lively intellectual development. Professor Tizard's
group found that well nourished children coming from 'high
stimulation' homes scored an average of 71.4 in an intelligence
test, compared with 60.5 for well fed children from 'low stimulation' backgrounds. The scores for children who had experienced (but recovered from) malnutrition were 62.7 and 52.9
respectively.

The interaction between inadequate nutrition and a poor
intellectual environment is all the more telling because the two
conditions tend to go together — making matters perhaps even
worse than they would be otherwise. Professor Cravioto
emphasises the importance of what he terms the children's
microenvironment, because he found that the homes of many
of his children with kwashiorkor were deficient in other ways
too. He discovered, for example, that the mothers of the
severely malnourished children listened much less often to the
radio than did those of healthier children. This could mean,
he argues, that those more interested in the radio were more

curious about the world and that this influenced their children. There is much more to learn about these subtle interactions.

It seems clear, however, that there are some 300 million infants in the world at the present time who are in danger of permanent, non-specific, brain damage because they are nourished inadequately during a critical period in their early life. The implication is that countries facing serious food shortages should seek to discriminate in favour of the under-twos.

A century after Pasteur

For World Health Day, on 7 April 1977, the World Health Organisation chose vaccination as its theme and promoted the slogan 'Immunise and Protect your Child'. Each year in the developing world over 80 million children are born who require — but do not receive — protection from diphtheria and other common diseases of childhood. Vaccines are, in a sense, magic bullets — specific prophylactic agents. Yet even here specific aetiology is left far behind, obscured by environmental, social, financial and political factors that at one and the same time make these diseases worse *and* interfere with the delivery of simple preventive measures.

Consider, for example, measles — a discrete infection caused by a particular virus and preventable by the corresponding vaccine. Despite this intrinsic identity, measles is for all practical purposes a different disease in the Third World and in the wealthy West. Rhazes (see p. 9), a Persian doctor who died in 1923, wrote the first known description of measles, in which he stated: 'Measles which are of a deep red and violet colour are a bad and fatal kind.' This form of the disease was rediscovered less than twenty years ago. In many developing countries it seems to be the infection that causes most deaths. Among malnourished children the mortality rate from measles is 400 times greater than in the developed countries. The more severe rash, as described by Rhazes, is a direct result of poor nutrition. The rash occurs not only on the skin but also on the lining of the mouth, the windpipe and the tiniest tubes in the lungs and the lining of the gut. So death is usually precipitated by pneumonia or diarrhoea. These complications are seen rarely if ever in Western countries. We are equally unfamiliar with the blindness frequently caused by measles in children already suffering a deficiency of vitamin A. It is poverty that turns the specific virus—one producing a substantial but rarely fatal illness in Britain or the United States—into a fearsome killer in Africa and Asia.

The other difference is that most children in the West are protected against measles, as they are against diphtheria, tetanus, poliomyelitis and other conditions, by routine immunisation. The reasons why the same vaccines are not deployed widely in the Third World are not medical. They are economic and logistical. To immunise a child for life against all of these common childhood infections costs an estimated two US dollars. Delivering the vaccines along the dirt tracks of Mozambique or their equivalent in other parts of the Third World can be a frustrating task. The problems of applying these unquestionably effective agents are thus those of conducting field operations in remote rural areas. Transport and fuel supplies have to be maintained and the vaccines must be kept safe and effective by refrigeration from the time they leave the manufacturing laboratory to the moment when they are given to children in the field. A 'cold chain' is required to ensure this safe transit. But in many rural areas the chain is still grossly inadequate, both technically and in terms of management, to keep measles and polio vaccines alive from manufacturer to child. From time to time epidemics of these infections occur among children who have been given the correct quantity of vaccine at the right age. What they have received, presumably, is material inactivated during its long journey. And, in urban areas, medical practitioners have been found demanding vast sums of money to immunise infants, often with vaccines that have lost their power of protection.

For these reasons the WHO is trying to convince member

countries that even limited local health services can be harnessed effectively to ensure that vaccines are delivered in good condition. Simple control laboratories can be set up to check their potency and safety. And, where it may not be sound economically to begin making vaccine from scratch, health services can halve their costs if they import concentrated vaccine and bottle it themselves. Measures of this sort could help to reduce the appalling gap between the 90 per cent or more of Western children who are immunised routinely against several potentially lethal diseases and the 10 per cent at most of children vaccinated in the less privileged parts of the world.

The WHO launched its Expanded Programme on Immunisation in response to a request from member states at the World Health Assembly in 1974. Its objective is 'to collaborate with countries in strengthening and expanding their health services so that they can protect their children by immunisation'. The target area for the programme comprises all children under the age of three, especially in rural populations and among the urban poor. The WHO provides aid but leaves management largely to local organisers who understand how best to promote immunisation in their areas. In Southern Mexico a Landrover moves from village to village, broadcasting the message: 'Come to the House of Health. Bring your children. Protect them against sickness. Come now to the House of Health.' And when the mobile team meets resistance from a *curandero* (traditional healer) it is as well that one of the team can speak the indigenous language and secure his co-operation. In Ghana, too, mobile field units, used to vanquish smallpox during the late 1960s, are now working as part of the campaign against other infections. The problem is that, whereas smallpox eradication was a once-and-for-all operation, control of other diseases will have to be maintained for the foreseeable future. In an area like northern Ghana, without roads and where one can walk for over an hour to reach a hamlet of a few huts housing less than fifty people, travelling on several miles further across country and streams before reaching the next habitation, the difficulties of regular surveillance are immense.

So while technical expertise is irreplaceable — in developing vaccines affording protection for longer periods, for example, and those better able to maintain their potency during travel — the tragic truth is that we already possess more than enough skill and knowledge of disease aetiology to confer life-long resistance on the 80 million children born each year who go unprotected. Dr Halfdan Mahler, Director-General of the WHO, singles out four reasons, none of them strictly medical, for the present sorry state of affairs. First, the public — and health professionals — do not appreciate the toll on health and lives taken by common childhood diseases such as measles and polio, or how effective immunisation can be. Second, health services are not in close enough contact with mothers to be able to reach their children with the right vaccines at the right ages. Third, there is a shortage of planning and management skill and field supervision needed for national vaccination programmes. Fourth, the cost of two dollars to protect a child for life may be more than the budgets of the health services of the poorer countries can carry.

A hundred years after Louis Pasteur began his experiments on the attenuation of chicken cholera bacilli — experiments which led to the introduction of vaccines against many other infections — vast numbers of the world's underprivileged children have not benefited at all. Those children, their resistance impaired by malnutrition, are as vulnerable as were the 'artificially' susceptible animals on which Pasteur achieved his dramatic historical results a century ago.

9
Beyond the magic bullet

When the World Health Organisation met in Geneva in May 1977 for the thirtieth World Health Assembly, delegates spent much of their time talking not about innovation in 'magic bullets' or the crying need to make specific therapies more widely available but about the vastly greater importance for health of developments in food production and living conditions. Dr C. Gopalan, Director-General of the Indian Council of Medical Research, warned the Assembly that malnutrition—not malaria or cancer or heart disease—could become the world's greatest single public health problem by the year 2000.

As Dr Gopalan pointed out, even the medical profession has not grasped the full magnitude of this problem. Chronic malnutrition—in contrast to sudden famine—does not produce dramatic or explosive situations and is rarely cited as the cause of deaths to which it contributes. Yet the number of sufferers from kwashiorkor and marasmus, which result from severe shortage of protein and calories, runs into several millions. Malnutrition is also potent in increasing susceptibility to infectious diseases and in aggravating their course (see p. 70).

At about the same time that the WHO was meeting in Geneva, four publishing events signalled what one hopes is a changing perspective on health and disease. First Dr Ronald Glasser, a paediatrician at the University of Minnesota, published his book *The Body is the Hero*, which demonstrated that man's own intricate physiological defences, evolved over a billion years, are infinitely more significant for the maintenance of health than are the tailor-made scientific weapons devised during the past century. The implication of this book, written by a specialist thoroughly acquainted with the merits of anti-biotics and high-technology medicine, is that doctors would do well to devote more of their energies towards understanding and encouraging the body's own capacities for self-restoration. On a broader scale, the appearance of the first volume of the new international journal *Culture, Medicine and Psychiatry* marked a growing recognition that sickness can be more fully understood by examining cultural factors in differing communities.

Then there were two reports, both published in the United Kingdom. The Office of Health Economics produced *Preventing Bronchitis*, which highlighted smoking, environmental pollution, and other social determinants of the disease and dismissed bacteria and viruses as its primary causes. Shortly afterwards the Royal College of Physicians launched a survey unambiguously titled *Smoking or Health* — contrasting with its two earlier versions called *Smoking and Health* which appeared in 1962 and 1971. This militant document warned committed smokers that every cigarette smoked, on average, reduced their lifespan by five and a half minutes, and called upon the British government to take drastic action to limit smoking because of its disparate and far-reaching effects on health.

We can conclude from these activities, and from the historical patterns traced in this book, that specific aetiology as an idea has had its day. The notion which has been as crucial to medicine as that of evolution in biology or the theories of relativity in physics is rapidly losing its power in helping us to understand or cope with the main diseases of today. This is not to say that we no longer need drugs or that we could dissolve these health problems miraculously by ensuring adequate food and sensible living for all. Formidable difficulties still remain. Dr Leonard Mata, from the University of Costa Rica, has pointed out that lack of food alone, for example, is not the only cause of malnutrition. 'Those who are familiar with rural

areas of developing nations are often amazed to find malnourished children in families where food is available in
amounts sufficient to ensure an adequate diet,' he writes.
'There may seem to be plenty of food in the house and, quite
strikingly, the mother of the malnourished child, as well as
other adults, may appear well nourished, or even overweight.'
Education of mothers in infant feeding and hygiene together
with numerous other domestic and cultural factors are
important here.

Even in the comparative affluence of Britain, a recent
survey of schools in the London borough of Brent showed that
DHSS guidelines for the composition of school meals were not
followed properly, 5 per cent of children were poorly fed, and
that the inadequately nourished among older pupils were
shorter in height than their colleagues. Poor purchasing, menu
planning and portion control were blamed for the inadequate
meals.

Similarly, exhortations by governments to smokers — or even
punitive levels of taxation — are not in themselves enough to
abolish the habit overnight. The RCP report found it necessary to call for a good deal more research into smokers'
attitudes towards their addiction and measures that might
help them to give it up. Acting to reduce the burdens of sickness stemming from malnutrition and smoking is vastly more
complex a proposition than the paper exercise of handing out
specific remedies to a population with particular afflictions.

Meanwhile, a substantial portion of medical research continues along its principal axis of specific aetiology. In some
areas, this may yet prove to be the correct approach. For
example, over the past decade many research workers have
claimed to have found specific microorganisms or chemical
aberrations responsible for various forms of arthritis. Though
none of these announcements has been vindicated, it remains
possible that a tidy explanation of this sort will prove to be
correct and that appropriate therapy can be devised. Perhaps
the problem in the past has simply been that of distinguishing
the particular cause against a complex background rather

than the inadequacy of the conceptual approach. For other conditions, the benefits likely to accrue from any discovery of an 'aetiological agent' are more arguable. Recent reports that a virus may be responsible for ulcerative colitis probably fall into this category. Should a microbe be implicated in the disease, it is unlikely that this will predicate the development of a corresponding cure. We know beyond reasonable doubt, though without great clarity (see p. 97), that emotional factors are important in precipitating colitis. They will scarcely be rendered irrelevant by the isolation of a particular component of the pathological process. More likely, such a discovery will parallel that of bacteria in bronchitic lungs (where they accompany and promote the disease rather than cause it single-handedly) or in carious teeth (where they play a significant role in eroding the enamel but are of little significance, compared with dietary habits, in measures to combat caries).

In his book *Genes, Dreams and Realities* the Nobel prize-winner Sir Macfarlane Burnet may have gone too far in denouncing molecular biology—which is now being pursued vigorously in the search for the most fundamental and specific therapies conceivable (see p. 60)—as of no significance for human welfare. Burnet argues that 'intrinsic' diseases and disabilities, ranging from cancer to the degenerative conditions that accompany ageing, are most unlikely to succumb to attempts to correct malfunctioning by tinkering with the genes responsible. He goes too far because it is likely that over the next few years the new discipline of genetic engineering may well yield answers to a number of hereditary conditions. Mutant or missing genes will probably be restored by incorporating into hereditary material in patients' cells the fully functioning genes necessary for health—a specific intervention akin to the administration of insulin to a diabetic. But the conditions amenable to this approach form a distinct and rare group. They are almost eclipsed by diseases for which this strategy would be irrelevant, unnecessary and ineffective. And the notion that molecular medicine could be harnessed to thwart the natural course of ageing is a cruel mirage.

Yet specific aetiology affords an unambiguous goal and promises a comforting certainty. Thus, the British Nutrition Foundation, in a publication reviewing the relationship of fibre to diverticular and other intestinal diseases, complains that 'dietary fibre has not yet been satisfactorily defined'. In other words, fibre should be analysed and scrutinised in the hope of finding a particular component that can be identified as active—and then presumably purified, packaged, and incorporated in foodstuffs in an exact, scientific manner. But the whole point about fibre is that it is *not* a specific element in food. Roughage is that invaluable 'non-digestible' portion that has been overlooked during past decades as nutritionists have identified particular classes of nutrients and categorised them chemically, each with its discrete role in metabolism.

Allied to a continuing faith in specific chemical therapies is an equally disproportionate belief in some quarters that particular organs in the body can be replaced by mechanical substitutes. The artificial heart is the outstanding example. Much of the research directed to that end is proceeding in the United States and the goal is a totally implantable, self-powered plastic heart designed to replace the natural organ when it has been ravaged by disease. Surgeons have, of course, been exploiting artificial devices for some time now in buttressing ailing hearts. They stitch in plastic valves; implant pacemakers in the chest wall to regulate the heart beat; and hook up heart-lung machines, outside the body, to take over the circulation during cardiac surgery. But as a product of science and technology, and certainly in terms of cost, a totally man-made heart represents an altogether different dimension. The technical barriers to be surmounted are immense and a successful prototype would be by far the most expensive gadget ever devised in the name of medical science.

The conventional attitude towards mechanical heart research is to applaud it as a proud symbol of sophisticated science and engineering ranged against one of our commonest and most crippling diseases. This orthodox view ignores four important considerations. First, even within the ambit of heart disease, there are far more sensible claimants for the massive funds now fuelling plastic heart development. These include studies on the prevention of chronic heart disease and on natural organ transplantation—always a sounder approach than mechanical substitution. Second, the financial and social problems of choice and availability that would arise should artificial hearts become available would be so great as to be insuperable. We have seen those difficulties on a relatively small scale in the case of artificial kidney machines—and have failed to solve them. Third, when we have evolved an effective method of preventing atherosclerosis—which will probably come not from medical science but from changes in diet or lifestyle—mechanical hearts could become worthless antiques overnight. Finally, and despite gargantuan investment, there are considerable doubts whether an artificial heart is a feasible proposition. Even the difficulties of fixing such a structure in place and of persuading the body to accept it—let alone making it work—are daunting in the extreme.

Dr Lewis Thomas is one of few distinguished radicals who see mechanical heart research, at the astronomical cost involved, as a gospel of despair. 'To be willing to invest the hundreds of millions of dollars that will probably be necessary for this one new piece of new technology almost demands of its proponents the conviction that heart disease represents an unapproachable, insoluble biological problem,' he writes. 'It assumes that the best we will be able to do, within the next few decades anyway, is to wait until underlying mechanisms of heart disease have had their free run, until the organ has been demolished, and then to put into the chest this nuclear-powered plastic-and-metal essentially hideous engine.'

There could be no more vivid contrast between the seductions of high technology medicine and the alternative approach that seeks to maintain health rather than to treat disease, to understand and then use the wider determinants of sickness rather than to cope with specific malfunctioning by individual therapies and replacements. It does not require

Ivan Illich and his *Medical Nemesis* to underline the irrelevance of such an elitist approach to medicine. Practising doctors themselves have begun to question the value of many of the tools that science and technology have placed in their hands — whether it be the sophisticated equipment used to maintain people as living vegetables in hospital after they have died in brain and mind or the antibiotics and other drugs that are prescribed so liberally. When a distinguished and well informed British general practitioner, Dr John Fry, talking of the £15,000 worth of medicines handed out annually by every UK doctor, confesses disarmingly that 'we must discover why all these expensive drugs are being prescribed and whether our patients' expectations and our own are being met', one realises that the everyday mechanics of medicine have got out of hand. Powerful nostrums, products of the modern pharmaceutical industry, are being dispensed in astronomical quantities but with little measure of their merits. What we *do* know, from various surveys, is that between 25 and 75 per cent of patients do not take their medication. The consequences of this failure, however, have not been delineated.

None of this should suggest that the drug industry is an anachronism which we could well do without, as argued by many of Ivan Illich's disciples. True, as Illich has pointed out, there is a large amount of iatrogenic disease in Western society — disease resulting directly from doctoring. True, the massive consumption of tranquillisers and related drugs is a scandal, a quasi-medical activity masquerading as precision therapy but in reality obscuring social, domestic and psychological tensions. True, many companies are guilty of pseudo-innovation, marketing products ostensibly as new, better and more specific cures when in reality the formulae differ little from those of their own or other firms' rival products. True, the expectations of patients have encouraged this bizarre trend — symbolised by a report which appeared in the *British Medical Journal* in 1977 describing a lady who was, literally, addicted to the idea of drug treatment. But we should remember that the industry *has* spawned innumerable remedies, from the penicillins to modern anaesthetics, which will continue to have invaluable applications throughout the world. What is drastically amiss is the notion that there is a specific drug cure for everything — a belief that has retarded our thinking about alternative approaches to health and disease.

Various surveys have shown that about 75 - 80 per cent of all patients seeking medical help have conditions that will clear up anyway or that cannot be improved even by the most potent of modern pharmaceuticals. In a little over 10 per cent of the cases medical intervention succeeds dramatically, by the administration of antibiotics, by surgical manoeuvres, or other specific measures. In the remaining 9 per cent the patients' troubles are diagnosed wrongly or treated incorrectly. They end up by becoming cases of iatrogenic illness.

What we have little numerical guidance on is the potential benefits derivable from non-medical, non-specific methods of preventing and treating disease. But there are powerful indicators. The Stanford Heart Disease Prevention Program has shown that health education efforts in two Californian towns were highly effective in reducing the risk of cardiovascular disease. Information on smoking, diet and exercise formed the main plank of the campaigns, which brought a 23-28 per cent improvement compared with a third town where no such crusades were mounted. The slight decline in deaths from coronary disease among middle-aged men in America and in Britain in very recent times also seems to have stemmed from increasing awareness of the factors responsible for coronary attacks, particularly smoking and lack of exercise.

We know, from work by Dr A. J. M. Brodribb at the Radcliffe Infirmary, Oxford, that a high fibre diet is effective in treating people with diverticular disease. We know that at least part of the explanation for the much higher infant death rate among American blacks, compared with white infants, is that more are born to teenage and unmarried mothers with low incomes. We have learned in Britain from Dr John Cohen that drug prescribing can be cut by some 25 per cent when marriage counsellors are available to assist doctors in helping the large number of patients whose problems are related to marital disharmony. And we know that smoking not only impairs smokers' health but may also damage a foetus before birth and increase the risk of respiratory disease among the children of smoking parents. Heavy drinking too, in addition to its relationship to alcoholism and cirrhosis of the liver, can harm the developing foetus.

Whether we look at the Third World or the industrialised nations, a greater proportion of ill health is determined by social, economic, domestic, and psychological than by specific factors. Its prevention devolves on changes in economic circumstances or personal behaviour rather than specialist intervention. In the developed countries, for example, many elderly people become senile for social rather than medical reasons; they are not cared for with the same affection and loyalty as are so many old people in, say, India or Pakistan. Conversely, in Asia, Africa and South America improved sanitation is infinitely more important to health than supplies of the newest antibiotics from the multinational drug companies.

As we have seen, the disproportionate emphasis of Western medicine on specific therapies has, as well as eclipsing the older, Hippocratic tradition, affected deeply the development of medicine in other parts of the world. Yet it has been the developing countries that, in recent decades, have begun to redress the balance through the evolution of community medicine and the use of barefoot doctors. Only in 1977 did the DHSS in Britain publish the results of a survey it had commissioned into the way doctors actually talk to the patients who come to their surgeries. And one of the key conclusions to the study, by Patrick Byrne and Barrie Long, was that medical practitioners 'display a remarkable inability to cope with anything but the most mechanical relationship with the patient'. More heartening is the fact that in very recent years the medical press has seen an increasing trickle of letters, papers and articles by doctors saying that they should have more time to exercise their pastoral role; to deal with grief; to mobilise their patients' own resources; and to discern and deal with complaints that are not organic at all, rather than to shower them with pseudo-scientific panaceas that at most mask their patients' symptoms and ensure that they do not return too quickly.

Much more research into psychosomatic aspects of disease is needed. Why, for example, do more men die in Britain on Mondays than on any other day of the week? The Office of Population Censuses and Surveys has shown that there is a consistently higher death rate from heart attacks on Mondays, possibly as a result of the stress of returning to work. We need to know more. Considerable resources also need to be ploughed into the study of ageing, not with a view to devising methods of retarding the natural process and prolonging the human lifespan (as urged by Dr Alex Comfort and others) but in the hope of combating some of the bodily miseries of old age. The recent establishment of a National Institute of Aging in the US, and plans for a similar body in Britain, may lead to valuable progress. Cancer research too appears to be moving into a more hopeful phase, with the investment, announced by the International Agency for Research on Cancer in May 1977, of 250,000 dollars to be spent over two years in a comparison of cancer in ten populations around the world. The basis of this investigation will not be laboratory searches for specific causes of malignant disease but an exploration of significance in occupations, lifestyles, cultural phenomena and environmental factors. Thus criticism of conventional medical research, founded securely on the concept of specific aetiology, should not lead us to dismiss research as valueless. A shift in the *style* of much research is needed. Investigators should concern themselves more with populations than with individuals, more with whole persons than with their individual organs or tissues, more with the mysterious interplay between mind and body than with the simplistic cause-and-effect model of disease.

Similarly, is it inconceivable that any society should seek to rid itself of doctors, as advocated by some of Mr Illich's followers, any more than medical practitioners will be replaced in the twenty-first century by computers—the prediction of

Professor Jerrold Maxmen. As a number of Third World countries have shown, however, primary medical care can often be
provided more effectively by auxiliary personnel working in
the community than by dispensers of specialist expertise living
apart. This is true too in countries like the United States and
Britain where social workers and even schoolteachers can have
a disproportionately greater influence than doctors on the
health of individuals and of the community. And it becomes
more apparent that the talents required of doctors are rather
wider than those that so many, by aptitude and training, have
today. As virtually all medical schools restrict admission to
students with high educational standards in science and follow
this by a training harnessed rigidly to the scientific approach,
it is hardly surprising that many of their products lack the
empathy and broader sensitivities that, in an average practice,
are in greater demand than detailed anatomical and physiological know-how. The undoubted successes of acupuncturists,
herbalists, osteopaths and other exponents of alternative
medicine also frequently bear witness to the failures of conventional therapy. Perhaps, as with the *rapprochement* between
the advocates of psychotherapy and of physical treatments for
mental illness, we shall see a growing tolerance (at least) by
scientific medicine of these heterodox disciplines.

The financial and political implications of the ideas
explored in this book are far-reaching. It is unquestionable
that greater reliance on pastoral care and a refusal by doctors
to deploy powerful chemical panaceas except when they are
genuinely needed could save vast sums in drug expenditure.
Mr David Ennals, as Secretary of State for Social Services in
Britain, has argued that the National Health Service would
gain about £2 million pounds a week if people stopped
smoking. In the Third World, the interplay between health
and economic development is one of the key political issues of
the day. Development requires a healthy population which, in
turn, can be secured only by adequate food supply and high
standards of environmental hygiene. Again, specific pharmaceuticals are not the primary consideration.

Given that the availability or otherwise of 'magic bullets' is not the central health question in any part of the world, and that most disease is related to habits and circumstances in a way that we understand clearly already, we are left with a dilemma. Do governments have a right to use authoritarian measures to ensure that their populations are healthy? Governments have long looked upon alcohol and tobacco as easy sources of taxation revenue. But increasingly they are beginning to raise for health reasons the financial penalties associated with consumption of these items. Should they, as in Norway, also seek to modify diet by financial incentives and disincentives? The treatment of lung cancer and coronary heart disease is expensive, so it is not unexpected that countries with health services provided out of the public pocket are showing the keenest interest in curbing ill health in these ways. But, whether we live in a democracy or under an authoritarian regime where state directives to maintain a fit population would be easier to impose, the temptation to go much further than exhortation and education to combat ill health seems certain to grow stronger.

Faced with the diminishing returns of research and medical care based on specific aetiology, we now recognise that, in the privileged regions of the world with their diseases of stress and affluence and also in developing countries where living standards are mediocre, the most urgent and far reaching choices in promoting health have little or nothing to do with scientific medicine. The economic and political decisions to be made in the light of this realisation are immeasurably more demanding than those taken in a world where the role of the doctor is simply to administer specific nostrums and that of the politician is to provide him with the means to do so. But then the real history of medicine has never been as simple as scientists have led us to believe.

Bibliography

The following list contains research papers and books I have consulted (including those specifically cited in the text) together with others that may be of further interest to readers.

Agnellet, M., *I accept these facts* (Max Parrish, 1958).

Anderson, E. S., 'The problem and implications of chloramphenical resistance in the typhoid bacillus', *Journal of Hygiene*, vol. 74, 1975, p. 289.

anon., 'Psychological factors in ulcerative colitis', *British Medical Journal*, 1 July, 1967, p. 5556.

anon., 'Smoking and disease: the evidence reviewed', *WHO Chronicle*, vol. 29, 1975, p. 402.

anon., 'Is grief an illness?' *The Lancet*, 17 July 1976, p. 440.

anon., 'Low spirits after virus infection', *British Medical Journal*, 21 August 1976, p. 550.

anon., 'Warning: smoking may damage your children's health', *British Medical Journal*, 7 May 1977, p. 1179.

Asher, R., *Richard Asher talking sense* (Pitman Medical, 1972).

Baird, D., 'Social research and obstetric practice', *Question*, vol. 2, 1969, p. 3.

Behar, M., 'A deadly combination', *World Health*, February-March 1974, p. 757.

Belloc, N. B. and Breslow, L., 'The relation of physical health status and health practices', *Preventive Medicine*, vol. 1, 1972, p. 409.

Bender, A. E. *et al.*, 'Feeding of school children in a London borough', *British Medical Journal*, 19 March 1977, p. 757.

Berg, J. W., 'Can nutrition explain the pattern of international epidemiology of hormone-dependent cancers?', *Cancer Research*, November 1975, p. 40.

Black, T., 'The baby who lived', *New Scientist*, vol. 69, 1976, p. 159.

Blythe, C., 'Eating our way out of debt and disease', *New Scientist*, vol. 70, 1976, p. 278.

Boyden, S. V. (ed.), *The impact of civilisation on the biology of man* (Australian National University Press, 1970).

Brodribb, A. J. M., 'Treatment of symptomatic diverticular disease with a high-fibre diet', *The Lancet*, 26 March 1977, p. 664.

Bulloch, W., *The history of bacteriology* (Oxford, 1938).

Burkitt, D. P., 'Epidemiology of cancer of the colon and rectum', *Cancer*, vol. 28, 1971, p. 3.

Burnet, F. M., *Genes, dreams and realities* (Medical and Technical Publishing, 1971).

Byrne, P. S. and Long, B. E. L., *Doctors talking to patients* (HMSO, 1977).

Campbell, G. D., 'Factors in the prevention of diabetes', *Prevent*, Vol. 1, 1972/3, p. 67.

Carter, C. O. and Peel, J. (eds), *Equalities and inequalities in health* (Academic Press, 1976).

Cartwright, A., *Human relations and hospital care* (Routledge & Kegan Paul, 1964).

Chandler, D. and Dugdale, A. E., 'What do patients know about antibiotics?', *British Medical Journal*, 21 August 1976, p. 422.

Cleave, T. L. *et al.*, *Diabetes, coronary thrombosis and the saccharine disease* (John Wright, 1961).

Coulson, C. A., *Science and Christian Belief* (Oxford University Press, 1955).

Cousins, N., 'Anatomy of an illness (as perceived by the patient)', *New England Journal of Medicine*, vol. 295, 1976, p. 1458.

De Kruif, P., *Microbe hunters* (Jonathan Cape, 1927).

Department of Health and Social Security, *Prevention and Health*, Cmnd 7047, 1977.

Department of Health and Social Security, *Prevention and health: everybody's business* (1976).

Diesendorf, M. (ed.), *The Magic Bullet* (Society for Social Responsibility in Science, 1976).

Dixon, B., 'Specific aetiology', *University of Durham Medical Gazette*, vol. 57, 1963, p. 124.

Dixon, B., 'Why do microbes misbehave?', *New Scientist*, vol. 51, 1971, p. 625.

Dixon, B., *Invisible allies* (Temple Smith, 1976).

Doll, R., 'The prevention of cancer', *Journal of the Royal College of Physicians,* vol. 11, 1977, p. 125.

Doll, R., 'Strategy for detection of cancer hazards to man', *Nature*, vol. 265, 1977, p. 589.

Draper, P. *et al.*, *Health, money and the national health service* (Guys Hospital Medical School, 1976).

Dubos, R., *Louis Pasteur: freelance of science* (Gollancz, 1951).

Dubos, R., *Mirage of health* (Allen & Unwin, 1959).

Farquhar, J. W. *et al*, 'Community education for cardiovascular health', *The Lancet*, 4 June 1977, p. 1192.

Feachem, R., 'Appropriate sanitation', *New Scientist*, vol. 69, 1976, p. 6.

Freeman, H. and Miller, H., 'Psychiatry and community health: a debate', *New Scientist*, vol. 53, 1972, p. 314.

Fry, J., 'Common sense and uncommon sensibility', *Journal of the Royal College of General Practitioners*, vol. 27, 1977, p. 9.

Gergely, J. and Baum, H., *Molecular Aspects of Medicine*, vol. 1, 1976, p. 1.

Gillett, J. D., 'Mosquito-borne disease: a strategy for the future', *Science Progress*, vol. 62, 1975, p. 395.

Glasser, R. J., *The body is the hero* (Collins, 1977).

Greenberg, D., 'A critical look at cancer coverage', *Columbia Journalism Review*, January-February, 1975, p. 40.

Harding Le Riche, W. and Milner, J., *Epidemiology as medical ecology* (Churchill Livingstone, 1971).

Halliburton, W. D., *Physiology and national needs* (Constable, 1919).

Harrison, P., 'Basic health delivery in the Third World', *New Scientist*, vol. 73, 1977, p. 411.

Haslemere Group, *Who needs the drug companies?* (1976).

Hinkle, L. E. and Wolff, H. G., 'The nature of man's adaptation to his total environment and the relation of this to illness', *Archives of Internal Medicine*, vol. 99, 1957, p. 442.

Illsey, R., 'The sociological study of reproduction and its outcome', in Richards, S. A. and Guttmacher, A. F. (eds), *Childbearing in its social and psychological aspects* (Williams and Wilkins, 1967).

Ingram, V. M., 'How do genes act?' *Scientific American*, vol. 198, 1958, p. 68.

Knowles, J. H., 'The responsibility of the individual', *Daedalus*, Winter 1977, p. 57.

Laing, R. D., *The divided self* (Tavistock Publications, 1961).

Lewin, R., 'The poverty of undernourished brains', *New Scientist*, vol. 64, 1974, p. 268.

Levi, G., 'Young lives at stake', *World Health*, July 1976, p. 20.

Liscowski, F. P., 'The barefoot doctor', *Eastern Horizon*, vol. 25, 1976, p. 20.

Maga, J. A., 'Influence of color on taste thresholds', *Chemical Senses and Flavor*, vol. 1, 1974, p. 115.

Marquardt, M., *Paul Ehrlich* (Henry Schuman, 1951).

Mata, L., 'Not just lack of food', *World Health*, May 1977, p. 25.

Maxmen, J. S., *The Post-physician era* (John Wiley, 1976).

McGlashan, N., (ed.), *Medical geography* (Methuen, 1972).

McKeown, T., *The modern rise of population* (Edward Arnold, 1976).

McKeown, T., *The role of medicine* (Nuffield Provincial Hospitals Trust, 1976).

McMichael, J., 'Prevention of coronary heart disease', *The Lancet*, 11 September 1976, p. 569.

Medawar, P. B., 'Is the scientific paper a fraud?', in Edge, D. (ed.), *Experiment*, (BBC, 1964).

Meyer, E. E. and Sainsbury, P. (eds), *Promoting health in the human environment*, (World Health Organisation, 1975).

Miller, H., *Medicine and society* (Oxford University Press, 1973).

Mills, A. R., 'The effect of urbanisation on health in a mining area of Sierra Leone', *Trans. Roy. Soc. Med. Hyg.*, vol. 61, 1967, p. 114.

Muller, M., 'Roche in the Third World', *New Scientist*, vol. 71, 1976, p. 326.

Muller, M., 'Lomotil: a case of moral incontinence?', *New Scientist*, vol. 73, 1977, p. 786.

Murray, M., *Guardian*, 29 December, 1976.

Murray, M. J. and Murray, A. B., 'Starvation suppression and refeeding activation of infection', *The Lancet*, 15 January 1977, p. 123.

Neu, H. C. and Howrey, S. P., 'Testing the physician's knowledge of antibiotic use', *New England Journal of Medicine*, vol. 293, 1975, p. 1291.

Nugrohe, G., 'Starting from scratch', *World Health*, April 1975, p. 26.

Office of Health Economics, *Hypertension, a suitable case for treatment?* (1971).

Office of Health Economics, *The health care dilemma* (1975).

Office of Health Economics, *Preventing bronchitis* (1977).

Penrose, L. S., *The biology of mental defect* (Sidgwick & Jackson, 1949).

Peters, E.-G. and Verhasselt, Y., 'Geocancerology', *Impact of Science on Society*, vol. 26, 1976, p. 311.

Pickering, G., *Creative malady* (Allen & Unwin, 1974).

Powles, J., 'On the limitations of modern medicine', *Science, Medicine and Man*, vol. 1, 1973, p. 1.

Rachman, S. J., and Philips, C., *Psychology and medicine* (Temple Smith, 1975).

Rice, T., *The conquest of disease* (Macmillan, 1927).

Rose, S., *The conscious brain*, (Weidenfeld & Nicolson, 1973).

Royal College of Physicians, *Smoking or Health* (1977).

Scrimshaw, N. S. et al., *Interactions of nutrition and infection* (World Health Organisation, 1968).

Sharp, C. L. E. H., and Keen, H., *Presymptomatic detection and early diagnosis* (Pitman Medical, 1968).

Shepstone, H.J., 'Radium the magic metal', in Crosslan, J.R. (ed.), *The Childrens New Illustrated Encyclopaedia* (Collins, 1946).

Sherrington, C., *Man on his nature* (Cambridge University Press, 1940).

Sigerist, H., *Man and medicine* (Allen & Unwin, 1932).

Silverman, M., *The drugging of the Americas* (University of California Press, 1976).

Simon, H. J., 'Ideas, germs and society', *Stanford Medical Bulletin*, vol. 19, 1961, p. 146.

Singer, C. and Ashworth Underwood, E., *A short history of medicine* (Oxford University Press, 1962).

Smith, H., 'Biochemical challenge of microbial pathogenicity', *Bacteriological Reviews*, vol. 32, 1968, p. 164.

Smythies, J. R., 'Recent progress in schizophrenia research', *The Lancet*, 17 July 1976, p. 136.

St Clair Symmers, W., *Curiosa* (Baillère Tindall, 1974).

Stewart, G. T., 'Limitations of the germ theory', *The Lancet*, 18 May 1968, p. 1077.

Sweet, W. H., 'Treatment of mentally intractable mental disease by limited frontal leucotomy—justifiable?', *New England Journal of Medicine*, vol. 289, 1973, p. 117.

Tait, I. and Hutchinson, E. C., *British Medical Journal*, 1 January 1977, p. 40.

Taylor, R. J. *et al.*, 'Use of bacteriological investigations by general practitioners', *British Medical Journal*, 13 September, 1975, p. 635.

Thomas, L., 'Have a heart', *Saturday Review*, January 1973, p. 52.

Thomas, L., 'On the science and technology of medicine', *Daedalus*, Winter 1977, p. 35.

Totman, R. *et al.*, 'Cognitive dissonance, stress and virus induced common colds', *Journal of Psychosomatic Research*, vol. 20, 1977, p. 55.

Tredgold, R. F., 'Effects of leucotomy on personality', in Ramsey, I. T. and Porter, R. (eds), *Personality and Science* (Churchill Livingstone, 1971).

Trethowan, W. H., 'Pills for personal problems', *British Medical Journal*, 27 September 1975, p. 749.

Vallery-Radot, R., *The life of Pasteur* (Constable, 1901).

Ward, R. R., *The living clocks* (Collins, 1972).

Watts, G., 'The ecology of hunger', *New Scientist*, vol. 69, 1976, p. 388.

Watts, G., 'What to do when the doctors leave', *World Medicine*, 26 January 1977, p. 17.

Watts, G., 'Guerillas as gurus', *World Medicine*, 23 February 1977, p. 61.

Wilenski, P., *The delivery of health services in the People's Republic of China* (International Development Research Centre, 1976).

Wilkinson, R. G., 'Dear David Ennals', *New Society*, 16 December 1976, p. 567.

Wilson, D., *Penicillin in perspective* (Faber & Faber, 1976).

Woodard, C., *A doctor heals by faith* (Max Parrish, 1953).

Index

smoking and health 67, 81-4 *passim*, 138, 139, 161, 163, 165, 166, 167, 183, 184, 187, 220, 221, 226, 227, 229, 230
Smoking and Health 220
Smoking or Health 220
Smythies, J. R. 116, 117
Snow, J. 68, 134, 187
social class and health 142-51
social factors in disease Ch. 6 *passim*, 227
social mobility 148-9, 154
social problems, medicalisation of 93-4, 96-7
socialised medicine 3, 6
Society for Social Responsibility in Medicine 85
'socioeconomic stress' 153-4
Solo (Java), self-help in 195-6
Spallanzini, L. 36
specialisation: Babylonian medicine 6; Egyptian medicine 5-6; undesirable effects of 88-91, 158
specific aetiology 1-4 *passim*, 21, 32, 35, 37, 43, 45, 46, 48, 54, 55, 57, 59, 60, 61, 63; causing unnecessary drug consumption 91-3; decreasing relevance of 220, 222, 224-5, 226, 227, 229-30; deficiencies as explanatory tool 64-87 *passim*, 96, 97; influence on mental illness 126; positive demerits of 127, Chs. 6-8 *passim*; specialisation encouraged by 88-91; undesirable effects of 88-95
specificity concept 18, 19, 35
spina bifida 163
spinal cord 8, 25
spontaneous generation 35-7, 39
'spontaneous remission' 103-4, 109, 113
Stahl, G. E. 17
Stanford Heart Disease Prevention Program 226
stethoscope 20, 21, 22
Stewart, G. T. 66, 69
stilboestrol 181

still birth, smoking and 83
Storey, P. 112
Strauss, E. B. 103
streptococci 53, 69
streptomycin 54, 78-9, 172
stress 81, 136, 163, 165, 228
Stress of Life, The 106
strokes 80, 161-2, 180
sugar consumption 144, 168-71 *passim*, 186
Suharjono, S. 209
suicide 152, 154
sulpha drugs 53, 76
sulphur dioxide 138
suppuration of wounds 41
surgery: antiseptics in 41, 73; survival after cancer surgery 86; undesirable effects of specialisation 88-90; wounds 41, 42, 73; *see also* appendectomy; brain surgery; heart surgery
Swammerdam, J. 14
Sweet, W. 124
sweetening agents 183
swine erysipelas 42
Sydenham, T. 2, 18-19, 35, 71
Symmers, W. St. C. 88
symptoms 20, 21
syphilis 10, 28, 52, 67, 69, 85, 115
Systema natural 20
Szasz, T. 114

Takimine, J. 58
taste, perception of 101-2
Taylor, R. J. 76
Taylor, S. J. L., *baron* 141
teaching hospitals 90
tetanus 48-9, 216
tetany 56
tetracyclines 54, 77
thalidomide 205
'therapeutic communities' 117
Third World First 210
Third World medicine Ch. 8, 229, 230
Thomas, L. 224
Titmuss, R. M. 149
Tizard, J. 214